PR

MW00989411

Motherhood Reimagined

"A beautifully written book about one woman's journey to have a baby on her own. It's an insightful and moving story that will inspire other women who face similar obstacles to becoming a mother. Well worth the read."
—**Jacqueline Mroz,** Contributor, *New York Times* and author of *Scattered Seeds: In Search of Family and Identity in the Sperm Donor Generation*

"Sarah has provided a gift to all women considering becoming a single mother with a beautifully written book that is both achingly painful and humorously honest. In her description of all that she had to go through to ultimately achieve her dream of having a child, her book reads like a novel that you can't put down. In the end, you realize that the peaks and valleys that she went through were in many ways a metaphor for life, one that she had no idea at the time would prepare her for her new role as a loving and patient mother."
—**Toni Weschler,** MPH, author of *Taking Charge of Your Fertility*

"In *Motherhood Reimagined*, Sarah Kowalski speaks to a generation of women who were told that they could have it all—only to discover that career success often comes at an emotional and physical cost. This honest, often heartbreaking, but ultimately uplifting memoir chronicles Kowalski's race against the ticking clock of infertility. The discoveries she makes about her body and mind translate into a compelling and poignant read . . . This book is a must-read for any women who hears the ticking of her biological clock."
—**Marika Lindholm,** CEO and founder of ESME.com
(Empowering Solo Moms Everywhere

"In the end, life dashed every expectation I had about how I would become a mother.' And yet, Sarah Kowalski did become a mother—just not in the way she had imagined. In this powerful, timely, and important memoir, Kowalski reveals how difficult it is to become a mother in your forties, and yet also how the journey has served as a beautiful and transformational process for her. Best of all, she helps anyone interested in becoming a parent who might be struggling with infertility, confused about reproductive options and technology, psychologically and emotionally distressed, and/or lost in the vast jungle of online information about IVF, adoption, sperm/ egg donation, and so on to navigate their way to motherhood. This book fills a gap in the literature on modern parenthood by offering wisdom, insight, and practical advice that will help you realize your dreams—one way or another."
—**Mei Mei Fox,** *New York Times* best-selling author and
   contributor at *Forbes*

"*Motherhood Reimagined* is a courageous journey through familiar life lessons. Using her embodied spiritual practice, author Sarah Kowalski faces her demons with vulnerability, humility, humor and insight."
—**Elena Brower,** author of *Art of Attention* and *Practice You*

"This very readable story of the author's journey to single motherhood by choice is a must-read for anyone contemplating becoming an SMC. It feels like a good friend is letting you join her on the trip as she shares her ups and downs, disappointments and celebrations. Informative, emotionally moving, and hard to put down."
—**Jane Mattes,** psychotherapist and Founder Single Mothers by
   Choice (SMC), author of *Single Mothers by Choice*

"Brave pioneers come in all sizes, shapes, ages and genders. Make no mistake, Sarah Kowalski is one of them. In her courageous memoir she opens up new territory, illuminating fresh possibilities for what it is to be an authentic dignified human being in the midst of probably the most profound life-changing event, becoming a mother, (in her case while being a single woman). She warmly, confidently and firmly draws the reader into the felt experience of all she faced, physically relationally, psychologically, financially and so on. Funny, inspiring, thought-provoking all at once. Sarah holds nothing back and opens up the chance for us to do the same in whatever we are facing in our own lives. A book for anyone living in our time and place."

—James Flaherty, author of *Coaching, Evoking Excellence in Others* and Founder of New Ventures West, Integral Coaching

"Get ready for an emotional and psychological journey. *Motherhood Reimagined* is a fascinating and intimate look inside the world of becoming a modern-day mother. An honest look at the emotional labor and physical challenges that arise on one woman's path to motherhood. Kowalski is relentless in her pursuit of becoming a mother, and grants us passage through her very own thick jungle of neuroses and tangles of self doubt while she bravely sharpens a machete of insight and truth to carve out her own path. A heroic and emotional journey that pulls you in and won't let you go until both the author and reader have found complete surrender."

—Madison Young, author of *Daddy: A Memoir and The Ultimate Guide to Sex Through Pregnancy and Motherhood*

"In the years that I've been communicating with Choice Moms, there are two things that stand out as true: 1) We don't realize how difficult it might be to conceive, which is exhausting to discover in our late 30s and 40s; 2) We underestimate our ability as strongminded women to "get it done," whatever it takes. Sarah is admirably able to openly capture both the vulnerability and the strength of her story of becoming a mother — a journey that never goes according to plan, and that teaches us more about ourselves than we can ever detail on our To Do lists."

—Mikki Morrissette, founder ChoiceMoms.org, and author of *Choosing Single Motherhood: The Thinking Woman's Guide*

"In *Motherhood Reimagined* Sarah Kowalski has accomplished what most memoir writers can never do. She has written two memoirs seamlessly woven together. One is an amazingly informative story about infertility and what one woman did to get pregnant. You will laugh and cry at Sarah's ability to capture the ups and downs of this saga. But she has also written a narrative about her spiritual struggles that is as interesting as her journey toward motherhood. This is one of those rare books that is not only replete with important information but it might even slip you onto your own path toward enlightenment."
—**Roy M Carlisle,** Senior Editorial Consultant, The Crossroad
   Publishing Company

"From the moment we meet Sarah Kowalski, a successful corporate attorney ignoring her biological clock, through her passionate quest to overcome infertility, to her early days of solo motherhood, one thing is for sure: nothing will go as planned. But Kowalski proceeds with determination, dissolving every physical and emotional barrier that dares stand in her way. This book is a must-read for anyone charting an unconventional path toward parenthood."
—**Cheryl Dumesnil,** author of *Love Song for Baby X: How I
   Stayed (Almost) Sane on the Rocky Road to Parenthood*

motherhood
REIMAGINED

Dear Eileen,
So happy to share this
journey with you.

XO,
Sarah Kowalski

A MEMOIR

motherhood
REIMAGINED

WHEN BECOMING A MOTHER
DOESN'T GO AS PLANNED

SARAH KOWALSKI

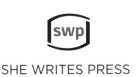

SHE WRITES PRESS

Published 2017
Printed in the United States of America
ISBN: 978-1-63152-272-7 pbk
ISBN: 978-1-63152-273-4 ebk
Library of Congress Control Number: 2017942207

Cover design by Elke Barter
Interior design by Tabitha Lahr

For information, address:
She Writes Press
1563 Solano Ave #546
Berkeley, CA 94707

She Writes Press is a division of SparkPoint Studio, LLC.

For Aiden

contents

part 1: remembering

part 2: struggling

part 3: arriving

dear reader,

*L*ike many women, I spent my late twenties and early thirties climbing the corporate ladder, kicking ass in my career. I worked hard—like sixty to eighty hours a week hard—and played hard, and I loved every minute of it. When a stress-related illness sideswiped my body and sidelined my career, I transformed myself from a corporate lawyer to a life coach, Qigong teacher, and healer. Back then, when people asked me (as they so often do ask women in their thirties) if I planned to have children, I waved them off. Maybe. Eventually. Someday. I'm not sure. Even as I edged into my late thirties, I felt no particular urgency to find a mate and start a family. As an educated, career-driven, young woman, with no potential long-term mate on the horizon, I'd been led to believe that it was no big deal to conceive a baby in my forties.

I couldn't have been more wrong.

And I am not alone. I regularly hear women lamenting how hard it is to find a partner and similarly lamenting that they waited so long to have a baby. For whatever reason—perhaps a misplaced belief in the power of modern reproductive technology, a plethora of celebrities who give birth well into their forties, and a lack of information about what it's *really* like to attempt pregnancy at a later age—they feel surprised and deceived when they learn that conceiving in your forties is not easy.

Like them, I learned the hard way. I woke up in my late thir-ties, partnerless, on the eve of perimenopause, longing for a baby, and fully aware that if I was going to become a mom, I was going to need to do it on my own. I launched Project Baby, tumbling down the rabbit hole of infertility options. Alternative treatments, Chinese herbs, western drugs, surgical procedures, IVF, sperm donors domestic and international, egg donors domestic and international—you name it, I encountered it.

My journey toward motherhood was an alternately harrowing, humbling, liberating, and even exalting trip that reminded me, time and again, that life rarely goes according to plan. In the end, life dashed every expectation I had about how I would become a mother. In fact, sometimes it seemed that everything that could go wrong did. But through the unfolding of unexpected circumstances, I was pushed to find learning in the hardship and to let go of my firmly-held beliefs so that something else could arise.

Along the way, my skills as a one-time lawyer came into play—researching options, weighing ethical concerns, strategizing to optimize outcomes, and negotiating with various players along the way. But figuring out the logistics of conception is only half the game. Because of my background as a life coach and spiritual seeker, I left no stone unturned when it came to clearing the path for conception—physically, emotionally, and spiritually.

My only regret—if it can be called a regret—about my journey is that it took so long. If I'd had a guide to walk me through the idea that it's possible and even simpler in some ways to raise a child alone, as well as the overwhelming information, logistics, and options for family-building, I would have saved considerable time and stress. If I'd had women to talk to—women who had walked this path before me, to share with me how they'd made the many decisions I faced, I would have moved more quickly through the process. If I'd had someone to work with who understood the emotional wrangling that comes with reimagining motherhood, I would have been spared so much time and heartache.

That's why I wrote this book—to offer a map to the women who come after me, to share the guidance and wisdom I gained in my struggle to become a mother.

We've all seen the pictures on the magazine covers: celebrities, happily pregnant (with twins!) in their mid-forties. But rarely do we see behind the scenes, into what they actually went through to get there. Rarely do women give voice to their journeys—instead they remain secretive, shamed by their body's inability. Consider this book the backstory—a real-life, messy-honest look at the journey from maternal ambivalence, to the courage to go it alone, to a no-holds-barred quest for pregnancy, to motherhood.

In it, I hope you find the inspiration, encouragement, and empowerment you need to find your own unique path toward motherhood.

I look forward to sharing my journey with you.

part 1: remembering

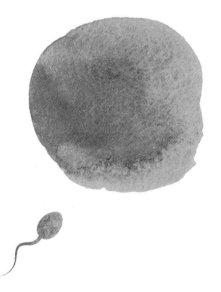

i always knew

I t was a warm, sunny West Los Angeles day in 1981. Whether summer or winter, the ocean breeze that graced the area gently drove the smog away and kept the temperature at an almost constant 70 degrees. I strolled down my block from the candy store, drinking my soda and sucking on some apple-flavored Jolly Ranchers, my usual after-school snack. As a ten-year-old growing up in an affluent area of LA called Pacific Palisades, I had few cares in the world. I waved to my neighbors, and I stopped to pet my friend's cat. Four doors down the block from my house, I noticed a new neighbor—a woman, probably in her late thirties, with a swollen belly. She had an easy, carefree air about her in her thin, purple, flowy, sleeveless shirt, Birkenstocks, and unshaved armpits. If I had known the word then, I would have said she was hippie-ish. When she glanced at me, I put my head down and kept walking, embarrassed.

Though to her my gesture probably said "shy," really I was plotting to befriend this very pregnant woman, not because she looked super cool (though she did), but because I wanted her baby. Yes, I was a ten-year-old baby-stalker, and thanks to my hypercritical mother, who had questioned my unabashed baby-lust more than once, I had begun to think there might be something wrong with me. So I kept my distance from my new neighbor, choosing stealth mode for the time being.

When I arrived home, I continued my after-school routine. First I watched an episode of *One Day at a Time*, then I did my homework. But fantasies of playing house with a real baby occupied my mind. I began strategizing how I could introduce myself to this baby mama.

That weekend, Operation Meet Mama commenced. First I played on my front lawn, staging elaborate weddings for my Barbies, after which they moved into my Barbie House and had many babies. When I got antsy, I moved on to gymnastics, practicing cartwheels and handstands, all with an eye on the house a few doors down. Even if she did come outside, I realized, it would seem a little weird if I suddenly rushed up to her the minute she emerged from her house. Clearly, I needed a plan that would place me directly in front of her house, so I could oh so casually say hello if she happened to, say, come out to get her mail.

Luckily, the stretch of road right in front of my new neighbor's house had recently been repaved, and that extra-smooth stretch of pavement had become the prime spot for roller-skating amongst the neighborhood kids. So I ran inside, grabbed my skates with the sparkly laces, orange wheels, and green toe stop, hunted for my special sparkly silver socks, which I had nicknamed my "Pizza-zium" socks, and geared up. Then I set out to roller-skate in front of her house, pretending to work on some tricks.

I followed this charade every day after school. It seemed like an eternity before I actually saw my pregnant neighbor again. But as soon as I caught sight of her, I looked away, pretending not to see her. *Ugh. Why did I do that?* But then, like iron filings to a magnet, my burning desire to play with that soon-to-be-born baby won over, and I made my move. "Hi," I blurted out as I paused my roller-skating routine and rested at the curb in front of her house. "How many months pregnant are you?"

"Seven," she replied. "It's my first."

Before I even found out her name was Sharon, I asked, "May I feel your belly?"

"Sure," she said.

I rolled over to her driveway where she was standing and

placed my hand on the gauzy fabric draped over her belly. I marveled at the hard, moving surface, astounded that there was a new life inside her. With Operation Meet Mama complete, it was time to launch my next offensive: I was gunning for the lead babysitter position in her household. Phase I of Operation Get Hired? I sat down on the curb, making myself comfortable, and started chatting, trying to sound like a responsible kid who a certain someone would like to have around after her baby was born. "I play with all the kids in the neighborhood," I bragged, regaling her with my baby expertise. Sharon seemed interested, so I began daily visits to her home, intent on sealing the deal. My fantasies of playing house with a real baby were quickly coming to fruition.

When the baby finally arrived, after two long months of anticipation, I was hovering, waiting for Sharon to return from the hospital. I doubt the new family was home for even five minutes before I bounded up their doorstep, asking to hold the precious little bundle. From that day forward, I became a constant presence at their house. In part, I hung out there because I preferred Sharon's company to my mother's. The two seemed polar opposites. For one, Sharon was much younger and cooler than my mom. But that was just the beginning. Sharon's relaxed attitude and bohemian style had a calming influence on me, especially in contrast to my mother's endless list of regimented ideas enforced by frequent yelling. I loved Sharon's creativity, like how she had given her baby the name, Sheriden, a combination of Sharon and Dennis, the father's name. My traditional mother, on the other hand, mocked this made-up name, calling it silly and odd. In fact, my mother mocked many of Sharon's choices—her unshaven armpits, her diet of raw, bright green produce that my British mother generally boiled into a drab green mush. Though I had connected with Sharon so I could play with Sheridan, unexpectedly, I had gained a surrogate mother for myself.

I'd spend hours talking to Sharon, recounting the most recent drama with the girls at school or which boys I liked. If I had tried to talk to my mom about this stuff, she'd lecture me, unable to hide her exasperation, "If Kimmy didn't invite you to her birthday party, then just stop trying to be her friend." But I'd been in class with the same twelve girls since kindergarten. My mother didn't understand the constantly shifting cliques and ever-flaring dramas were inevitable. She just wanted everything to go smoothly, and my distress stressed her out. Talking to Sharon, however, made me feel grown up. I could unload my feelings without fearing judgment, and I could trust her opinions and advice.

Every day, I would rush home from school, have a snack, do my homework, and run down to Sheriden's. Sharon would sit at her kitchen table, shelling beans or folding laundry, and I'd chat with her while chasing Sheriden around the house. I took care of everything for Sheriden—fed her, changed her diapers, kissed, and cuddled her. I loved Sharon, but I also loved this baby and wanted to spend every possible moment with her.

After nearly a year, my mother and Sharon agreed to let me babysit Sheridan. I was only eleven, so it took some negotiating. But I'd been taking care of Sheridan while Sharon was home practically every day for her whole life, so obviously I knew what I was doing. At first, I'd watch her for only a few hours at a time, and only if my mother was home to call upon if anything went wrong. But before long, I'd reached my goal: I was Sheriden's main babysitter. Not only was I thrilled to get to play house all on my own, I was getting paid $4.50 an hour for it! When Sharon had a second baby, I was doubly happy to watch both Sheriden and her little brother.

For as long as I could remember, I had known with all my heart that, more than anything in the world, I wanted to grow up and be a mother. When anyone asked how many children I wanted to have, I'd say, "Eleven." I obviously knew nothing about what raising a gaggle of children entailed, but my devotion was clear. Loving and caring for Sharon's children deepened my resolve to keep children in the center of my life. I was single-minded about it. Until I wasn't.

forgetting

I f my child self had peered into a crystal ball to see her future, she would not have recognized the corporate lawyer sitting in a swanky San Francisco bar with her friends, sipping a $15 glass of Zinfandel. I had continued to follow my interests in all things maternal, creating summer camps for the children on my block, babysitting throughout high school, studying women's reproductive rights and medical anthropology in college, and writing my thesis about the medicalization of childbirth and breastfeeding in an urban aboriginal community in Australia. Though I had toyed with the idea of a career in academia, I'd chosen law school instead, hoping to make an impact on policies related to maternal health. I focused my studies on women's autonomy over their bodies, especially during pregnancy, and I even interned as a patients' rights advocate.

Upon graduation from law school, however, I realized that the jobs I longed for at such places like Planned Parenthood or NARAL (National Abortion and Reproductive Rights Action League) often required a pro-bono stint and/or proved so low-paying that I'd never pay off my student loans. Meanwhile, the dotcom boom had law firms heavily courting new hires, and the high pay and prestige of Silicon Valley pulled me off track. I compromised, accepting an offer at a firm with a health law department and an impressive roster of biotech clients, telling myself at least I would get exposed to interesting bioethical questions.

So here I was, thirty years old, a corporate litigator exchanging extraordinarily long hours for generous compensation. In my off-hours, I tried hard to prove to myself that it was all worth it by indulging in lavish dinners, buying expensive wine, shopping to my heart's content, and traveling to exotic and expensive locales. Somewhere between my rocket-speed career and my jet-setting single life, I'd completely lost my resolve to have children. Though we'd all been warned about "golden handcuffs" in law school, the ridiculous figures we began earning right out of school had lured us. We'd assumed we'd be able to walk away when we were ready. I, for one, thought I could not be bought long-term.

Meanwhile, though, I could be found frequenting trendy downtown bars like this one, where my friends Joanie and Collette, whom I had known since college, and my coworker Tania had just ordered a second round of drinks. Then someone lobbed a million-dollar question to the group: "Do you guys want children?"

My closest friend and sidekick, Tania, blurted, "NO WAY!" exhaling her cigarette smoke. "I would never give up my freedom. And children are brats." This didn't surprise me, coming from my adventure buddy. Together, Tania and I had shaken off bad break-ups by escaping to Cuba to learn salsa dancing. Back home, we became obsessive salsa dancers, working late at the law firm, until the clubs heated up, then dancing well past midnight, then crashing for a couple hours before dragging ourselves back to work at 9:30 A.M.

Tania wasn't like other people I'd met in college and law school, who were more conventional in their choices and lifestyle. She was incredibly intelligent, gorgeous, confident, and committed to having an interesting life and that meant no kids. I looked up to Tania in many ways, including her negative attitude toward children, and realized only in retrospect that it subtly seeped under my skin and into my psyche. She woke up something inside me that had partially died in law school. She, and salsa dancing, helped me rekindle passion and excitement when law seemed to be trying to suck me dry.

Joanie, the youngest of eight siblings, jumped in next, "I definitely want kids. And I don't see why it has to be a choice between children and a career," she said raising her glass. "You can always figure something out." I believed this about Joanie. As our resident Superwoman, she seemed always to juggle a million commitments with grace. She'd worked in Africa as a raft guide, written a guidebook on Mexico, and competed—on weekends, while balancing her job at the California Attorney General's office—in pro divisions of mountain biking and snowboarding. If anyone could find a way to blend parenthood and career, Joanie could.

Colette, meticulous as always in her Banana Republic sweater set and tasteful diamond earrings, shared her plan. "I want to be married by the time I am thirty-three and have children no later than thirty-five." Then she joked, "And let's throw in the white picket fence," suddenly conscious of her absurd specificity. "But really," she continued, "I've started Internet dating, and I intend to go on one date a week until I meet my husband."

Ugh, I thought. Internet dating, a new trend at the time, was taboo to me, something I'd assumed only serious losers would do. So Colette's revelation surprised me. She was cool and fun and not desperate. She was just . . . goal oriented. She knew what she wanted, and she was going to make it happen. Still, when I thought of online dating, I recoiled. No, thank you.

Now all eyes turned to me. "Do you want children?" Joanie asked.

Completely detached from my childhood baby-lust, I churned up a non-committal half-answer. "It depends on who I end up with," I said. "I can't answer that question until I meet my partner. Then we will decide together."

"Well, so then what's going on in your dating life? Anyone special?" Joanie pressed. Everyone's eyes lingered on me, as if they expected some sort of big confession.

"No," I said. "I saw Jason the other week. He's still blowing me off. I know he's struggling, and he says he's not ready for a relationship, but he's such a good guy and so hot." My secret plan? To spend more time with Jason, so he'd realize how incredibly cool I was and how compatible we were. This was my pattern: 1) Get hung up on a guy who claims—for one reason or another—he's "unavailable." 2) Hang around until he realizes his mistake, which he never did.

Honestly, dating and relationships had never come easy to me, and I'd spent years at a time being single. Instead of recognizing that I needed to get back in the game quickly, I'd either pine too long or reject perfectly good mates for silly, superficial reasons. I wasn't willing to admit that it was time to get over it and get serious about finding "the one." But now that my friends and I were approaching our mid-thirties, the peak fertility window, I could sense that most of them had a clear goal in mind: get married and have kids. It was the driving force behind much of what they did. Somehow, I didn't get the memo. I kept flitting around, fickle, uncommitted, and—I would later realize—refusing truly to focus on finding a partner, for fear of seeming desperate. Instead, I focused on cultivating a fun-filled, interesting life.

A few months after that conversation at the bar, Joanie announced that she was getting married. Colette and Lori, my closest friends from college, were next. Then a cascade of friends from college and law school announced their marriages and subsequent pregnancies. Of course I was happy for my friends, but I was also starting to get worried. For one, I was losing my party buddies. But, more importantly, I was beginning to wonder about my lack of serious relationships. Why did partnership continue to elude me? Despite my growing curiosity, I never admitted, not even to myself, how badly I wanted to be partnered. Instead, I acted as though I was okay being single. I continued to follow the age-old advice, "Do what you love and the right person will show up." I kept up my busy social life, but the partnership I longed for never materialized.

Meanwhile, my certainty about motherhood had vanished, replaced by a strange mix of ambition, fear, avoidance, and circumstance. In my mind, "Do you want children?" was a question for a couple to answer together, not one for me to answer before I met my partner, or, God forbid, for me to consider as a single woman. Rather than exploring the question for myself, I deferred it for a later time, repeating that motto, "I can't decide until I meet my partner, then it will be a joint decision."

a dramatic shift

A few months after my friend Joanie had announced her engagement, I woke up with a neck ache and a dull pain in my right hand. The previous month, I had billed close to three hundred hours, so a little physical tension made sense. But the symptoms grew. I tried to accommodate them, using the mouse with my left hand to relieve the pain on the right, and procuring a standing desk so I could change positions regularly. Weeks passed, and these changes did little to curb my pain, which worsened every day. Then one afternoon, as I sat at my desk, looking out the windows of my fancy downtown San Francisco office, I shook my nearly-numb hands, trying to revive the sensation. Suddenly, a strange, electric tingling traveled from my neck, down my arms, into both hands, terrifying me. Something was seriously wrong, and I needed to find out what it was.

Soon after, I was diagnosed with a repetitive strain injury called thoracic outlet syndrome (TOS) and chronic fatigue. I pushed on through the pain at work, leaving regularly for various physical therapy appointments. Despite my efforts and reasonable accommodations from my law firm, four years of pushing my limits, long hours, stress, pleasing others, and rising to the top had taken a permanent toll on my body. After a year of trying to make it work, I left my position as a litigator and filed for disability.

Many of my friends distanced themselves, disturbed that a competent, smart woman could spiral downward so quickly. Others refused to believe the intensity of my pain. "But you're always in a good mood," they would say. If I had acted grouchy, would they have expressed more empathy?

"I can barely wash my own hair," I explained to one. "I have to lower my arms to take a break to get the blood flow back into my arms when I lather the shampoo." With another I shared, "I can't open my front door because I don't have the grip strength to turn the key in the lock." But just as many friends stepped up with essential support, helping me with grocery shopping and even household chores I struggled to do, like laundry and cooking. With a friend who shared my Polish American ancestry, I joked, "I don't think I'll ever be able to open a jar of pickles again." She knew a pickle-less life was sad prospect. Luckily, I had help with those stubborn lids.

My dating life took the worst hit. In the cutthroat, driven, success-oriented Bay Area, stepping out of the career race at the height of the dotcom boom dropped my sexy quotient significantly. The woman I was—passionate, forward moving, insanely busy in my work and social lives—had disappeared. On a handful of first dates, describing my current life, I felt the words fizzle as they left my mouth, landing on the table with a thud. How could I convey any excitement or vivacity? I left each date feeling ashamed and boring, the exact opposite of the image I had been cultivating for years. For the time being, I gave up my hope of finding a partner and, because the two were inextricably linked in my mind, any thoughts of having a child. Who knew if I would ever be able to lift a child, much less support one financially on my meager disability compensation? My biological clock continued its relentless ticking, but I wasn't listening.

As my social life quelled, my healing odyssey began. I sought help from all manner of healing arts—acupuncture, cranial sacral, biofeedback, massage, and Pilates. Many days, I'd have two appointments in a day. I'd spend the rest of my time doing the exercises designed to help me get better, including walking as much as possible to improve my circulation and keep the blood flowing to my hands.

Healing didn't stop with my physical body, though. I had to say good-bye to my identity as a self-sufficient lawyer with a full and active life. I could no longer bike, ski, or snowboard much less cook or even grocery shop. Slowly, I realized that so much of who I thought myself to be was tied to my activities and interests. With those taken away from me, I had to grapple with what I wanted to do and be in this world. All my life, I had been surrounded by people who lived by the motto, "Work hard and play hard." Both my parents and the culture at large had taught me to value a conventional, ambitious career path. But my body—and perhaps with it my spirit—refused to keep up. What would give meaning to my life now? I was in a free fall. It would be years before I could see my law career as a divergence from my original calling—my interest in health, healing alternatives, and maternal wellness.

Eventually, I would come to see this stripping away as an incredible teacher instructing me in one of the central tenants of Buddhism, the concept of no-self. Only when the ideas, interests, pursuits, and thoughts I had grasped onto in order to create an identity—or self— were stripped away, could I understand that none of them were me. From a worldly perspective, this experience of no-self looked like a scary void. Yet in that void I could recognize my true nature, my essence. In the end, I would see my illness as a homecoming to the nature that wanted to be expressed. But at the moment I couldn't see further than the physical pain that had me in its grip. I was forced to address my immediate concerns rather than question the purpose of my life. I didn't know yet that my quest for physical healing would lead me right to the center of the life I was meant to live.

Even though I treated my recovery like a full-time job, I saw very little improvement in those first few years, until I attended a Feldenkrais Awareness Through Movement Lesson (ATM). On a studio floor lined with students lying on thick blankets, I followed the instructor's lead through a detailed body scan. Then I rolled from my back to my belly, raising my arms above my head on the ground in front of me, Superman style. I'd then side bend, bringing my left shoulder and pelvis toward each other. "Notice what happens to the arms and legs resting on the ground as you side bend," the instructor said. "Do they remain still or do they move?" I'd been so focused on the curve of my ribs and spine that I hadn't noticed that one arm lengthened and one arm shortened in response to the movement of the spine. I alternated, curving my spine and pelvis from one side to the other, thereby moving my arms and legs. The whole group of us moving like this—we looked like a bunch of lizards slithering along the ground. I was blown away by the power of this movement, so subtle that it felt almost like I wasn't doing anything, yet it created such a noticeable effect. By the end of the session I was captivated. I *had* to learn more.

As my fellow students streamed out of the studio, I eagerly approached the trainer to share my experience. I felt taller and more relaxed than I had in ages. "That was amazing. I haven't been able to lift my arms above my head without pain in several years. I've tried acupuncture, Pilates, biofeedback, massage, cranial sacral, and more, but nothing has eased my pain until this moment."

"That's great," he said. "It's likely because this lesson reminds students that the arms are powered by the pelvis. I've seen this many times. People with repetitive strain injuries have cut off their arms from their core and they use the arms like appendages tacked onto the body."

"Yes, exactly," I nodded enthusiastically. "How can I learn more?"

"There's a four-year training program starting next week," he told me. "You should come."

That was all it took. I enrolled as soon as I got home.

The following week, I attended the first ten days of the four-year training program at Fort Mason Center in San Francisco, a space where exposed industrial pipes and low-pile carpet were offset by a wall of picture windows overlooking the bay. The eight-hour day alternated between Awareness Through Movement (ATM) lessons and Functional Integration (FI). During ATM lessons, we were most often laying on the ground, guided to sense subtle movements in our bodies, while following verbal instructions from the trainer. The movements were simple, like rocking my pelvis back and forth or from side to side, or lifting one arm into the air above our heads, while noticing which part of the body pushed into the ground and which raised up.

Each of these lessons featured a reference or baseline movement, something we could come back to intermittently, to see if we noticed any changes in our range of motion or if our sense of ease was shifting throughout the lesson. We might be asked to turn around to see behind us, noting how far around we could turn with ease. Then we would be directed to do other movements that could be thought of as smaller components of the reference movement, like shifting weight on the hips, twisting the ribs, or rotating the head. By directing awareness to the smaller components, the body was tricked into recognizing aspects of the reference movement that may not have been evident before. Almost always, this type of exploration lead to greater ease, range of motion, and gracefulness when we returned to the reference movement.

During an FI lesson, the trainer demonstrated movement with a student, gently touching and guiding the student's body to move in ways that highlighted the movements we'd been verbally guided to do throughout the ATM. In this way, we were honing our ability to see movement and clarify it, so we could sense it more clearly in our own bodies when we returned to the movement in an ATM lesson.

Throughout the day, the trainer, who sat at the front of the room, kept saying, "It's not about whether you succeed in doing the movement or moving farther, but rather about the quality of your awareness as you do the movement. Can you notice when you clench your jaw or hold your breath, even when you are doing a simple movement like raising your arm?" With this guidance, I was awakening into a different way of being, where success and achievement were based on an internal quality of ease, as opposed to getting something done or pushing myself to do more. The method constantly reminded me to notice the temptation to sacrifice ease and pleasure just to feel a sense of accomplishment, in this case performing the furthest extreme of a movement. On the outside, it looked like I was doing a body practice, but on the inside this training was challenging my deeply held beliefs. It was sneaky and profound, and it began to reduce my pain like nothing else had.

On the seventh day of the workshop, I arrived tangled up in financial stress. How was I was going to survive? Now that I was starting to see improvement in my body, I worried that my benefits might be discontinued. The irony that feeling better could put my financial lifeline at risk threw me into a panic. How I was supposed to recover if any small improvement might jeopardize my disability benefits? My thoughts spiraled out of control, spawning visions of chronic couch surfing and homelessness.

During the Awareness Through Movement lessons that day, we focused on softening the ribs and chest. As I checked in with my body, I noticed that my shoulders had dropped what felt like several inches. My chest was soft and felt malleable. I could feel each breath expand my entire torso cavity, down to the perineum. I could also feel all of my ribs—front and back—as well as my low back moving. With each in-breath, my shoulder blades gently glided across my back. My mind filled with the image of a large paper bag, rhythmically inflating then deflating with each out-breath. It occurred to me that I'd been freezing my ribs in a static position, habitually impeding my breath. My ribs, especially those in the back, likely hadn't moved in years, a common symptom of stress and long hours of computer use. At the same time, my fear had dissolved, replaced by a sense that I would figure it all out if I just took it one day at a time. Even when I tried to conjure up panic-inducing ideas, they simply would not stick. In their place, I felt safety and support. My mental state had transformed completely. I was amazed. My circumstances had not changed one bit, but my outlook had, all because I released the pattern of anxiety in my body.

❧

At some point during the training, Chris, a soft-spoken, slightly dorky English man with a receding hairline, sat beside me to watch an FI demonstration. I was fidgeting, wriggling from one position to another, trying to get comfortable. Chris, a fellow student in the training, and I had already become friendly, spending lunches together and strolling along the waterfront. He had told me that he was a Qigong instructor, but I was too embarrassed to admit to him that I had no clue what that meant. I had shyly pretended to know and quickly changed the subject. Noticing my fidgeting, Chris leaned over and whispered in my ear, "You are in pain, aren't you? I could help you." Before I could respond, he waved his hand behind my back between my shoulder blades. "You have a sharp pain right here, don't you?" I nodded. *How did he know?* That was the exact point.

Even though he wasn't touching my back, I could sense exactly where Chris's hand was at any given time, almost as if he were reaching inside my back with a whisper-like touch. *What is that? Am I imagining that?* As I tuned in, I felt a cold sensation leaving my body, like a gentle wind flowing out of me. I felt immediately lighter, calmer, and more peaceful. Within a few minutes, my pain was alleviated completely. I was baffled.

After the demonstration, I asked Chris, "What was that? What did you just do to me?"

"It was a form of Qigong treatment," he explained. The cold sensation was something called Binqi, which translates as "stale Qi." It could be cold, itchy, or even prickly, and it causes pain and discomfort. Chris had been trained to sense it and remove it from the body. His teacher, who worked at a hospital in China, did these treatments as a matter of course. Nothing unusual in Chinese culture, yet Binqi was one of the most magical things I had experienced to date. "You should come to my class sometime," Chris offered. "I can help you get out of that pain."

I still didn't know what Qigong was, but I took note.

෨

After my experience with Binqi, I was intrigued by Chris, and within a few months I found my way to one of his weekly classes, held in a little studio attached to his house in the hills of Mill Valley. There, I found ten other students chatting in small groups. Chris was not yet in the room, and I did not recognize anyone. My nervousness started to mount, until a small group of students turned to welcome me.

"How did you hear about the class?" asked a woman in her early thirties with dark hair and a big, bright smile.

"I know Chris from the Feldenkrais training," I explained.

"Oh, right! He told us you might be joining us. Welcome!" she beamed, making me instantly feel more at ease. After a few more pleasantries, a skinny blonde woman blurted out, "We make a lot of noise during practice, but don't be freaked out. Just ignore us." I didn't know what she was referring to, but I nodded and smiled.

A few minutes before class was scheduled to start, Chris entered from the adjoining house, wearing khaki cargo pants and a plain T-shirt, carrying a cup of tea. He immediately came over and gave me a big hug. "What have they been telling you about class?" he asked. "Don't believe anything they tell you," he joked. I was starting to wonder what in the world would happen.

When Chris took his place at the front of the room, he transformed from a casual, self-deprecating guy into a man who gently commanded attention with his clear presence. He stood simply, no posturing or grandeur, but effortlessly powerful. In his proper British accent, he directed us to stand quietly. "Just sense your body. Don't do anything," he said emphatically. I felt myself drop into a state of awareness that I had not experienced before. He directed us to shift our weight from our left to right legs, while noticing the pattern of pressure that traveled across our feet. These instructions were familiar, akin to a Feldenkrais ATM lesson.

"When you feel the most stable, where is the majority of your weight across your foot?" he asked, giving us time to explore and notice. "Imagine drawing a line between the second and big toes down the length of the foot. Can you place 50 percent of your weight on either side of that line? How stable does this make you feel?" I immediately noticed how much more stable I felt when I weighted my body as Chris had suggested. This orientation forced me to load through my leg in a way that made me feel solid and balanced. Upon this adjustment, my whole system seemed calmer. A stillness washed over me. I inhaled deeply, noticing the sense of relief that came with my breath.

For another fifteen minutes, Chris continued guiding us to notice small details about our bodies. I marveled at the minutia I had never been aware of before, even though I'd been training in Feldenkrais for a few months. "Now, start to bring the majority of your weight onto the ball of your foot. Avoid the temptation to lift the heel up as you do this. Experiment with the idea of taking the heel down and back toward the floor as you tip your weight forward more onto the ball of your foot," Chris instructed. "You may start to notice that you have to change the posture of the entire body to make this possible. You must do something in your low back to make this happen. Can you tell what it is?"

I had noticed, while trying to follow Chris's directions, how I had bent my knees and tucked my tailbone under slightly, causing my low back to lengthen gently, as opposed to its usual arching.

"The posture is like you landed after jumping or dribbling a basketball," Chris explained as he bent over slightly and mimicked dribbling. "Try it. Try jumping and landing. Notice how you land." He explained this was the position we were looking for, because it lowered the center of gravity in the body to the area in the belly just below the belly button called the dantien, considered the center or pump of the energetic body and meridian system.

How cool is this? I marveled. I had never even heard of the dantien, but as soon as we were instructed to draw our attention to it, most of the students in the room started yawning or burping. Some even started singing or chanting. So *this* was the noise they'd warned me about.

Chris answered the question I held in my mind. "Because the

dantien is the powerhouse of the energetic system, people will start to have reactions when the center of gravity hits there. It's as if we are literally kicking the dantien." As he spoke, he wandered around the room, waving his hands in front of various students, which seemed to intensify or exaggerate whatever the student had been doing before. When he waved his arm in front of the blonde woman, who was now humming a beautiful tune, she sang even louder. As he approached someone who was swaying a bit from front to back, he made a quick sharp movement with his hand in the air in front of the student, who then started moving back and forth quite rapidly and burst out laughing. The laughter was contagious, spreading to others around the room. I expected them to quash their laughter like obedient students, but they continued. Chris smiled and carried on. Obviously, there were no rules in this light-hearted class. I felt even more welcome. I could get used to a life like this.

Chris explained, "Qigong is about developing what're called internal forces. If you were training in martial arts, you would cultivate these forces internally and learn how to apply them externally to hurt your opponent. In Qigong, we use these forces to improve health and open up the body's energetic pathways. When I wave my hands in front of a student, I link to their dantien and Qi and help open the pathways or meridians more fully." We did a standing practice, in this position, for another thirty minutes before we sat for meditation.

The meditation format was unfamiliar. As we sat at the edge of our chairs, unsupported by the backrest, we did a mini Feldenkrais lesson to notice some aspects of how to sit effortlessly. Then we imagined that we were sitting on a lake and could see our reflection. I placed my mind on the reflection and imagined the body sitting on the chair was slowly melting, filling in the image in the water below us. I focused easily, feeling increasingly present, like my being was married to the ground in a way I had never experienced before.

At the end of class, Chris sat back in his chair, his warm brown eyes sparkling. "I'll give you a few minutes of theory. Any more than that and I'll not only confuse you but also bore you to tears." I appreciated his teaching style—he acted dismissive, like nothing special was going on, but I was taken aback by the remarkable experience I'd just had. I was anything but bored, and my analytical mind wanted to know *everything*.

Chris introduced us to the three aspects of the practice— physical/biomechanical, energetic, and mental/perceptual. "These three pillars of practice are always interrelating and influencing each other," he told us. "The biomechanical study allows the energetic system to come alive in our perception. Once we wake up the energetic system, we can start to notice shifts in our mental habits and changes in our perception." I would later understand that this constant attention to all three systems was what made Chris's teachings unique. But as we ended class that evening, I felt confused—many of the intricate instructions had gone over my head, and I was still unsure why other students had been making sounds during their practices. Rather than being turned off or intimidated by this confusion, a common experience amongst people new to Qigong, I was intrigued. More importantly, my pain had reduced significantly, and I was again able to hold my arms over my head for a full minute. Also, I felt clearer and calmer, less anxious. I was hooked.

I soon learned that Chris, this unsuspecting, humble, and gentle man, was not only a powerful Qigong instructor, but a somatic genius and an all-around profound healer. In his quest for authentic, deep knowledge, Chris had moved around the world, studying various disciplines. In his early twenties, he traveled to India for a few years to study yoga with a master there. Later he traveled to a Buddhist center in Thailand to study with a great master, then to a sacred valley in Tibet to study Tibetan Buddhism. He'd studied closely under three Qigong masters for several years, and at other times had taken on in-depth studies of martial arts, shiatsu, acupuncture, anatomy, and Feldenkrais. He knew more about the history of the disciplines he had studied than anyone I had ever met. With this extensive training and twenty years of teaching and treating students, Chris had synthesized his learning into his own system. Though he called himself a

Qigong teacher, I would always call him my Qigong master. But even that label does not come close to explaining the depth and breadth of what he teaches and embodies. Through Chris, I would find the physical healing and the spiritual guidance I craved.

resurfacing the question

I n 2010, seven years after that first Qigong class, I was a new woman. I'd finally let go of my identity as a lawyer and admitted to myself that I would never return to corporate litigation. I was so taken with my early experiences of Qigong that I strived one day to attain the status of Qigong Master. I knew it had taken Chris over fifteen years of training to call himself a teacher, but I wasn't intimidated by that. I wanted to start down that path. After about four years of practice with Chris, he gave me permission to teach classes in his system of Qigong, and he agreed to continue mentoring me as a teacher.

Meanwhile, I'd earned certifications as a Feldenkrais practitioner and an Integral Coach. I'd gone back to work, launching my own coaching business based on the Embodied Clarity Method (ECM), a coaching modality I developed, which combines the rich philosophies of Moshe Feldenkrais, Integral Coaching, and Qigong.

Although I was still experiencing pain, I could relieve the bulk of it by practicing Qigong daily and limiting my computer use. I still couldn't work full time, and there was no way I would earn a salary commensurate with my litigator's paycheck, but with the support of disability benefits, I could work part-time and give my body the rest and attention it needed. Coaching proved the perfect option for me, because it required little computer or desk time, and I could flex my schedule as my health allowed.

But more importantly, I loved the work. Many of my clients were standing at a crossroads I recognized. They were high achievers, rushing toward burnout in careers that no longer fed their souls. My coaching approach highlighted how their bodies played an important part in their mental wellbeing, their ability to get things done, and their ability to be perceived positively by others. Using the principles I had discovered in the early days of my Feldenkrais training and had rediscovered through my years of Qigong study, I helped my clients calm their anxiety (or any other distressing emotion) by undoing the muscular pattern associated with it. Some of my clients wanted to adjust their relationships to their work. I taught them how to rest on the supportive structure of the skeleton so they could feel more grounded, less frazzled, and ready to set appropriate boundaries instead of reacting in the moment. Other clients wanted to explore new directions in their careers and their lives. I helped them learn to soften their rib cages or otherwise settle their bodies and thus their minds. In this way, they could stop the panic and become present to themselves and their deepest desires. Alternately, I drew attention to and released habitual contractions, giving them a break from their habitual experience of themselves and opening up an opportunity to try on a new orientation to the world and to themselves.

The deeper I moved into coaching, the more I recognized this work as my true calling. I had always been drawn to issues surrounding health because in my heart, I wanted to be a healer. I could explore my fascination with health and healing not as an academic study or as a series of legal policy issues, but in the trenches, helping people understand their bodies, specifically the links between their thoughts, emotions, and physical sensations. I made this connection while working through the exercises in Julia Cameron's *The Artist's Way*. Cameron explains that many people step off their true path because they are afraid to *be* the artist, actor, healer, or other creative type. Instead they pursue a more conventional, stable career that skirts the thing they wish they could be. This described my career path precisely. I had studied Psychology and Medical Anthropology, which analyzed and compared various healing systems, because academics, policy, and ethics had been acceptable career choices. Never did I register that I actually wanted to *be* a healer because that path stretched too far outside the realm of what I'd been taught, by my family and my culture, to consider reasonable.

As my pain became less of a threat to my day-to-day existence and as my work came into alignment with my physical abilities, I started to reconsider my self-imposed dating hiatus. But before I stepped back into the dating pool, I had some junk to clean out of my psyche, to make space for a healthy relationship. I recognized that my relationships with my parents had affected my dating dynamics in the past, so I asked Chris to support me as I delved into those issues. I worked hard to fully forgive my parents for the wrongs I perceived in my upbringing. I let go of the need for their approval by, among other things, letting go of Sarah the lawyer and embracing Sarah the Qigong teacher and coach, amidst their vocal disdain for my new choices. Having never felt fully accepted and unconditionally loved by my parents, Chris helped me release old messages so that I could believe I was worthy of love and relationships. It was painful but powerful work, and after several years of introspection, I felt emotionally healthy and ready for a romantic relationship.

With some of the deep family wounds healed and a new career gaining momentum, I felt my Qigong practice deepening. Having learned how to address most of my physical ailments, and gotten my life largely on track, I was ready to go deeper in my practice. And that meant, uncovering more and more about my own essence. This aspect of the practice, often referred to as a prenatal practice, focuses on returning to your nature before you were embodied. I was ready for it.

During one session, as I lay on a low, wide treatment table, Chris gently lifted my head and cradled it in his hand. I was lying on my back, my knees propped up to support my back and reduce as much muscular tension as possible. As he gently held my head in silence, he made micro-movements that helped me let go of even more tension and created a wonderful floating sensation. I drifted in and out of a strange dream-like state, blissed out and calm. Then his voice, calm and gentle, jolted me out of my daze, "You are going to be forty next year, if you want to have children, you better get focused and get on with it."

I practically jumped off the table in shock. But I remained in place, calming myself, letting Chris's words penetrate my being. He was right. I was thirty-nine, and while I felt ready to date, a serious romantic relationship seemed a distant dream. As long as I held tight to my mantra, "I'll decide if I want kinds once I find my partner," becoming a mother seemed an even more remote prospect than finding a perfect mate.

Chris's words looped in my mind for the next few days. The baby question was all I could think about, really. Initially, I resisted. *Thirty-nine is not that old*, I thought. *Women are having babies later and later in life. It's a myth that you can't have a baby well into your forties*, I argued to myself. *I have time to hold out for a partner. There's no rush!* But another part of me percolated on his words. I knew I needed to focus on this question. If I wanted a baby, I needed to get deliberate about finding a partner so we could get pregnant as soon as possible, or I had to think about having a baby alone. Both options sounded like bizarre, foreign concepts to me.

As I sat in my gynecologist's cold exam room, awaiting her arrival, I decided I'd use this routine visit as an opportunity to ask some preliminary questions about my situation and late-in-life pregnancies in general. Perched on the vinyl table, covered only by a thin sheet of paper and a hospital gown that didn't close in the back, I tried to keep my back relatively upright despite the absence of a backrest, something I always did to prevent back and neck aches. But with my feet dangling off the table, the dreaded stirrups pushed off to the side, it was hard to find any ease—with my posture or my looming questions. Still, when my doctor entered the room, I broached the topic. "I'm thinking about having children," I told her, "but I'm not ready yet." I noticed I was fidgeting, and I made a conscious effort to stay grounded by feeling into my body and breathing down, imagining I was sinking into the ground. "Are there any tests I can do to get a sense of my body and how long I may remain fertile?"

After she ran through some questions about the regularity of my (very regular) cycle, she suggested, "You should test your Follicle Stimulating Hormone levels," she told me. "That will give us an indication of how hard the body is working to ovulate and thus some idea of the quality and quantity of eggs someone may have." On her way out the door, she handed me a lab slip.

A few weeks later, my levels came back normal. Nothing to worry about at this point, but something my doctor had said during my appointment rang in my ears, "This number can change next month. Just because this number is normal now does not mean it will be normal tomorrow." Though her words were stern, her demeanor was calm and relaxed, so I figured this was just a little speech she gave to all her patients facing the baby question in their late thirties. So I felt no urgency. Many of my close friends had just had their first or second babies at forty. No one around me was having trouble getting pregnant, at least that I knew about. I assumed I had time.

dating at 39

Since the baby conversation with Chris, I was no longer oblivious about my desire to have kids. Finally it was seeping in: to make children a reality, I needed to find the right guy soon. The news about my healthy ovaries confirmed my plan: to date with intention to mate. By this time, online dating had become the norm, and something I had done on and off over the years. But I was ready to kick off my renewed online search for love. Sitting in my living room, armed with a big glass of wine to take the edge off, I signed up for a Match.com account.

From the outset, every question I answered seemed to narrow my dating pool significantly, particularly the kid question. My options included: have kids, don't have kids, wants kids, don't want kids. I nervously rapped my fingers on my laptop, wishing "I'm waiting to decide until I find my partner" would appear. I stared at the two options: "wants kids" or "don't want kids." I took the leap: I checked "wants kids," slugged a gulp of wine, and moved on.

Next came describing the kind of guy I was looking for, and honestly, I was having a hard time figuring that out. I was torn between two worlds—the more conservative, conventional world of my lawyer days, and the more open-minded, adventurous one I lived in now. In recent years, I'd gravitated to more bohemian friends who, like myself, were interested in spirituality, meditation, and healing, as well as music and dancing. But I still valued the focus and drive that characterized the lawyer life. I didn't live entirely in either world, and in many ways the two stood at odds with each other.

I spent probably too much time agonizing over my profile, trying to strike the right balance of level-headed and professional, mixed with unconventional, kind-of-out-there on the spiritual/ healing front. Before logging out, I fired off some emails to a few guys who seemed interesting. I wanted to sound witty and smart, but something about communicating with a profile sapped all my creativity. Most of my emails felt stiff and—I feared—a bit desperate, coating me in a residue of embarrassment. *How do people do this?* I wondered, closing my laptop for the night.

A few days later, one of the most promising men I had emailed, responded, "You seem amazing, but I want children. At your age, that's tricky, so I am going to pass on meeting you." Ouch! Why didn't he just stab a dagger into my heart? Of course, Mr. Wrong was highlighting a truth I was loathe to recognize: my fertility was waning quickly. But who actually *says* that? I could see this as a red flag indicating this man wasn't a great catch. Ideally any man I would fall in love with would be willing to take me as is—warts and old age and all—even if it meant a long, difficult, or even impossible road to parenthood. But over time, more men responded with similar sentiments, and I could taste nature's bitter irony: the men who wanted kids as much as I did wanted women younger than me.

On the flip side, my inbox was continually flooded with inquiries from men in their fifties and even sixties, who deliberately overlooked my designated age range, thirty-five to forty-five. Who were these lurkers? Were they preying on women who had passed their fertility window, assuming we wouldn't care about dating much older men? Even worse was the guy who reported he was forty-three, but as soon as I saw him, I knew he had lied. Sure enough, within a few minutes, he confessed he was in fact fifty-three, but "young at heart" and "in really great shape." So much for trying to date someone even within five years of my age.

I wasn't the only woman in the Bay Area struggling to find men my own age to date. A brief survey of my personal landscape showed that many of my male friends were dating women ten to fifteen years their junior. Maybe they didn't want to feel rushed about the child thing, or they wanted a trophy girlfriend, or they did it just because they could. As for the women my age? I knew several amazing single women, but we all agreed, the list of available men was painfully short.

Who knew online dating at thirty-nine could be so difficult? After several months and quite a few dates, no one piqued my interest. Sure, I could get all revved up about the ultra-sexy, bad boys, but the men who would make a good baby daddy? No spark. As for the men's perspective, it broke down like this: if they wanted kids, my age was a ticking time bomb signaling that I would need to rush through all the normal stages of a relationship in order to get to the kid part right away. For those who did not want kids, because I'd checked that damn "kid" box, no one believed I was open to casual dating. No matter which way I sliced it, my age was forcing me into an "undatable" zone.

In an attempt to sidestep the online world entirely, I decided to up my opportunities to meet someone organically, getting involved with organizations and activities that touted personal awareness, spirituality, and open communication as their foundations. But more and more I was finding that many of the people involved in these groups were practicing polyamory. One guy in particular typified this trend. I met him at a friend's party, a gorgeous African American man with dark, silky skin, bright eyes, and a devilish smile. We gravitated to each other instantly, and I was on top of the world when he confidently asked me out.

He invited me to choose the restaurant, and I picked a hip seafood joint in the Mission District, deemed a great first date place because it was not too expensive, had great wine by the glass, and was never too crowded or loud. As we sat across each other, we engaged in a quick, smart, playful banter. I learned that he'd found some success through a start-up, he seemed emotionally and financially stable, and he was *hot*. As I was taking a sip of my second glass of a Syrah, feeling encouraged so far, he confessed, "I have something to tell you."

I paused mid-sip. *Uh oh, here it comes.*

"I have a girlfriend, but we are in an open relationship." He paused just briefly before continuing, "I've already told her that I will be having sex with you tonight, and she's okay with that."

I almost sprayed my sip of wine across the table. *What?* So many parts of what he'd just said were so wrong, I didn't know where to start. His assumption that we'd be having sex? Or the fact that he was flirting heavily with me while his girlfriend sat at home waiting for him. Internally, I slammed on my brakes, bringing the date to a screeching halt. But instead of walking out immediately, I turned on the anthropologist in me and asked him some questions. How did this set up work? He explained that he used to just cheat on his girlfriend. But now, instead, he told her of his plans beforehand, and his girlfriend could dabble too. "My only requirement is that I talk to the guy before my girlfriend gets physical with him," he explained innocently. "The only time she was interested in someone, he declined after she asked him to talk to me."

Are you kidding me? Yes, when I stepped out of the law firm, I left my more conservative self behind, and yes, polyamory was a Bay Area phenomenon at the time, so much so that *San Francisco Magazine* had run an entire issue dedicated to it. But I was still quite conservative in wanting a committed relationship with one man. My date's arrangement did nothing to change my opinion.

I was starting to suspect my mad dash to find a partner willing to make babies with me wasn't going to work. It was easy to get lured into continuing to find a partner, *I'll just try a few more months*, I could hear myself say. But when I was willing to be completely honest with myself, I knew it wasn't going to happen in time. Still, I wasn't ready to put down the idea of a committed relationship, but I was losing hope. Disillusioned by the dating scene, I started to wonder if I should just get knocked up by some hot guy on a vacation. I had always had a love of Italian men and culture. More than once, I fantasized about going to Italy for a month or two seeking a hot romance that would hopefully produce a love child. But that would mean unprotected sex with a virtual stranger. And worse, I couldn't get around the deception. I'd have to decide whether or not to tell my fantasy lover, and if I did tell him, I'd have to convince him that I did not need him to be involved in parenting our child. That sounded more than messy, like I'd be bringing a child into the world with a dark cloud looming over our heads.

I eventually got distracted from online dating when I met Rodrigo, a tall, handsome man, with a sinewy body I loved. Initially he swept me off my feet, complimenting me constantly and taking me seriously as a healer, something I couldn't say about my family or even some of my friends. He was completely present with me, dedicated to being an amazing lover. He was separated from his wife, and he already had two kids. I was totally smitten by the time I realized he was still hooked into his ex emotionally, rendering him unavailable for anything serious. I was so enjoying our exciting dates and his careful attention, though, I was not willing to give it up. Instead, I told myself it was okay to have a frivolous relationship. Even though he did not want kids, or even a girlfriend for that matter, it was perfectly okay to have fun for fun's sake. Predictably, I flip-flopped a bit along the way, occasionally reverting back to my old habit of thinking I could win him over, but eventually I settled into this casual arrangement. In theory, it allowed me the freedom to keep looking for a more serious relationship, but in reality I was no longer giving off the available vibe. Because I wasn't yearning for companionship, my dating efforts faded.

My connection with Rodrigo sparked a new idea—a man did not have to be both my boyfriend and my baby daddy. The person who satisfied my romantic, emotional, and physical cravings did not also have to be the father of my child. My various needs and desires—for emotional support, physical intimacy, companionship, baby-making sperm, and parenting support—didn't have to be met by one person; they could be met by different people. This concept was equal parts revolutionary and eye-opening. I wasn't ready yet to take the leap into parenting alone, but this idea put an enormous crack in my conventional thinking, opening up endless possibilities.

trying to decide

T hroughout my last-ditch effort at dating, Chris continued guiding me through my practice, helping me get in touch with my essence, unveiling my true path in this life. By now, I felt the urgency to decide whether I wanted a baby. Since dating wasn't going so well, that meant deciding whether I wanted to have a baby alone. "I'm here to help you uncover what direction you want to take in your life and help you clear out the confusion and misperceptions as they arise so you can see clearly what you want," Chris had explained. If a child was part of that equation, I needed to make that choice before I ran out of time. At the time, Chris was renting office space from a friend across the bay, so I'd make the trek down to see him every few weeks.

During one session, we began seated in chairs, facing one another in the dim office with a dark cherry wood desk in one corner and Chris's bodywork table in the middle of the room. I gave Chris an update on my dismal dating life, joking about the absurdity of my encounters. Then he cautiously broached the baby topic. "Well, you could just have a child alone. I know you've been toying around with the idea, but it's time to start thinking about it more seriously," he cautioned. "I think you could do it alone if you wanted to. You are finally getting stable enough."

Chris was right. I finally had my feet on the ground financially. I'd been in a big battle with my private disability company for the past several years. During that time, they had refused to pay me. When the case settled after several years, they were required to pay me a lump sum in back payments, allowing me to put a down payment on a home in Oakland. Emotionally, after years of concentrated healing work, I was feeling more and more settled. Though Chris had sensed that my nervous system was "very delicate and easily disturbed"—in other words, supremely sensitive to my surroundings and my own emotional ups and downs. I'd been learning how not to get knocked off balance as well as how to return to myself in the face of difficult situations.

"But," I interrupted, "I don't know if I *want* to do it alone. I'm not even sure I want to have a baby." Immediately I could hear it: the whiny tone in my voice. I launched into my list of things I still wanted to do in my life that were likely impossible if I had a baby. "I still want to spend a year in India studying, healing, and singing." My voice began shaking. "I won't be able to go back to Cuba or go out dancing." I went on and on, complaining about the independence and freedom I'd have to give up, while Chris sat at the end of his chair, his back effortlessly straight, nodding his head.

His feet rested squarely on the ground in front of him, his legs bent at a ninety-degree angle. I recognized this posture. It was something I did with my own clients. Chris was creating a physically neutral state in his own system, so he could tune into me and track changes in my nervous system—my breathing, my eye movements, the color my skin, my neck tension, or my overall posture. I knew that Chris would notice when I started to lose my ground, and would understand my feelings beyond my words. If I remained neutral while speaking, he knew there was "no juice" behind what I was saying. If, in contrast, my breathing became erratic or I tensed my neck muscles, he could tell I was getting into a hot topic, one that raised a surge of emotion.

When Chris held this state, my experience was akin to sitting down in front of a giant mirror. Nothing I said could stick to him. It was as if my thoughts or concerns bounced back at me, or instead just fizzled in midair. Often I went into my sessions with Chris armed with an agenda—a long list of topics to discuss. But as soon as I sat down in front of him, I either couldn't remember the items on the list, or they no longer felt that important. Other times, because Chris was able to maintain a neutral stance, he could reflect my current emotional state back to me, which in turn amplified my feelings. Often, in the face of this reflection and amplification, I'd burst into tears as soon as I started speaking.

"I'm not sure I want to have a baby if I have to do it alone," I said. I could remember how badly I'd wanted children when I was younger, but my rational adult mind dreamed up every reason under the sun to avoid motherhood. "I'm afraid I'll end up single forever if I have a baby alone. Who wants to date a woman who already has kids?" I implored. This fear of remaining single forever loomed over me. I was adamant that no man would ever want to be with me if I already had a child. In my search through online dating profiles, I myself had eliminated men who already had kids. Even before online dating, in my early thirties when my girlfriends and I talked about whether or not we'd date a guy with kids, the consensus was, *No, too much baggage.*

In fact, when I considered my mantra, "I won't know if I want kids until I meet my partner," I realized it had risen out of a similar fear of rejection. I was afraid of scaring men off if I showed that I was committed to having a child. Having never known any boys who were obsessed with babies, I assumed that most men were somewhat indifferent to having children. Women were the ones who really wanted kids, right? When I thought about trying to date as a single mother, I assumed that a man would be unmotivated to raise a child that was not his own flesh and blood. And that man, whoever he was, would have to fall in love with both of us. The dating equation already seemed difficult enough without adding a child into the mix. At the time, I could only think of one male friend who had married a woman who already had kids. I blame twelve years of Catholic school for coloring my view about dating with children.

"Will I even be able to date again if I have a kid?" I asked Chris.

"You might be freed of dating forever," Chris laughed. "You did start this session with a list of the dating horrors." I loved the way he and I could banter with each other. It helped lighten my mood. But I also knew on a deeper level that Chris had a plan, and his irreverent joking was helping me break down my barriers to see the absurdity of what I was saying.

"And, how will I support myself?" I continued.

"I don't worry about you financially," Chris said reassuringly. "You're very smart, and you know how to make money."

I paused and tried to articulate what was coming up for me next, but it was having a hard time coming out. I held my breath, fighting back tears, a lump stuck squarely in my throat. "But what if I can't have a baby?" Now tears started to stream down my face. "What if I can't do it alone?"

"Why don't we lay you down now," Chris said, motioning to the table.

As I nestled in, Chris placed huge pillows under my knees and a small, flat pillow under my head. "Are you comfortable?" he asked.

I took a huge breath and nodded yes.

Chris began making small adjustments to my body, putting his hand under various ribs, and then waiting. I took a big breath without needing to be prompted. Then he made some adjustments to my pelvis, sending a gentle force through my spine and into my head. With each adjustment, I grew more relaxed and calm, settling more and more into the table. The chattering in my mind faded into a quiet stillness.

After a few moments, Chris spoke gently, "So, the list of rational reasons not to have a baby is long. But what does your heart yearn for?" And then, chuckling a little, he continued, "No one would ever have a baby if it was a rational decision. Can you shut off that lawyer mind of yours for a minute to listen to your heart and gut?"

Chris's voice calmed me, yet when he asked what I wanted in my heart, I held my breath and that telltale lump formed in my throat. I tried to hold back the tears. It was futile. Tears dripped out of the corners of my eyes, rushing into my ears. "I'm so confused," I managed to say. "I don't know what I want."

I wasn't sure why I was crying. At the time, I thought the confusion upset me. Eventually I would understand that Chris's words had touched some deeper part of my knowing. The mere mention of my heart's desire stirred something, connecting me not only to my purpose but also to regret for not yet living that purpose. "That's okay," said Chris reassuringly. "Don't worry. It will become clear. For now, just rest." He continued the session, in silence. Chris is a firm believer that the nervous system cannot learn when it's overloaded. I took the cue and allowed myself to let go of the incessant internal debate over whether to have a baby. I did not need to figure it out in that moment. I trusted that my subconscious mind was chewing on the equation and that the best thing was to allow my body and mind to get clear and calm so that a deeper knowing could surface. As Chris worked on my body, my mind got quieter and quieter. A familiar blissful, dreamlike state came over me.

By the time I left the session, I felt peaceful and content. As I drove home, I turned on the radio and sang along to the carefree pop tunes that played. Everything looked particularly beautiful to me. I marveled at the expanse of the bay as I crossed the Dumbarton Bridge. The salt evaporation ponds on the Hayward side of the bridge shone their glorious mix of deep clay red and burnt umber. I was no clearer on the baby question, but the list of concerns I'd rattled off to Chris at the beginning of my session seemed distant and much less important.

Over the coming weeks, the internal debate would kick up again and again, my lawyer brain squawking away. I couldn't hear my heart's voice over the din. It's surprising to look back now and see how far removed I had become from my maternal longing. Had I lost my longing to become a mother, or had the fears about doing it alone clouded my desire? I was no longer ignoring the baby question, but still, I could not decide.

frozen eggs and embryos

I n April 2011, a few months after my fortieth birthday, I had another routine visit with my OB/GYN. Time to ask more questions about my options for having a baby. Apparently a partner wasn't going to materialize, so I needed a Plan B, in case I decided to green light the baby option. The prospect of using a sperm donor freaked me out, and my list of reasons for not having a baby alone hadn't changed. But I recently, I had heard about egg freezing. Maybe that could buy me more time? I wanted to know more.

As my doctor performed my pelvic exam, she confirmed that I could indeed freeze my eggs for later use. However, the technology was still new at that time and pregnancy rates were so low that she considered it virtually useless. "It's still considered experimental," she said, a note of apology in her voice. "And the odds of getting any good eggs are extremely low in your forties." I was a bit taken aback by her bluntness, but I also appreciated her honestly. "It also means you will have to go through IVF, with all the drugs to hyperstimulate your ovaries."

Hormones, drugs, and a low success rate? I balked at taking Advil, let alone birth control pills. IVF drugs were definitely out of the question for me.

She continued, "I'd advise that if you were going to retrieve eggs, you should fertilize them and freeze embryos instead.

Embryos are much more viable and much more likely to survive a thaw." She paused, took a deep breath, and proceeded somewhat cautiously, "But of course, you'd need a sperm source to do this. So, if you don't have a partner, that means using a donor." She knew she was hitting a nerve. I held back tears as I managed to choke out, "If I had a sperm source, I wouldn't be in this predicament in the first place."

While I acknowledged that using a sperm donor was a useful option for some people, I recoiled at the thought. Though I couldn't have articulated it at the time, I feared using a sperm donor said something about me—that I was a horrible failure because I couldn't find a partner who wanted to have a child with me. I was also suspicious of a sperm donor's motivation to donate. Did they have some ego complex driving them to spread their seed in the world? Plus, I was conflicted about the idea of not knowing who the biological father of my own child would be. From my unexamined, uninformed perspective, at that time in my life, it seemed foreign, sad, strange, and scary to purposefully have a child with no father.

Then there was the freezing of the embryos. I'm not particularly religious, but I am spiritual, and I believe in reincarnation. Fertilizing a bunch of eggs and then freezing them in time—to me it would feel like I was violating of some universal law, though I couldn't articulate what that was. I didn't judge the practice of embryo freezing as immoral, but I did view it as potentially confusing to the natural order of things, and I wasn't sure I wanted to mess with that.

From a more practical standpoint, I knew research had shown that embryos and the resulting offspring were unaffected by the IVF process. But I had reservations about whether there was enough data. In Vitro Fertilization dated back to 1977. Was that enough time to confirm the long-lasting effects of the process?

Over time, I would arrive at a place where none of these concerns mattered anymore, but as I sat in my doctor's office that day, making a baby alone felt impossible. "I can't get over the idea of freezing my future baby," I explained to my doctor, "so it looks like I'm stuck with finding out how my own eggs are faring and deciding what to do based on that information."

The doctor laid out a plan, "Okay, let's just test your FSH levels again so that you can see if there is any urgency right now."

"My cycles just started to be irregular in the last few months," I explained. I had also noticed that I had gone from constantly wiping an oily glisten from my face to slathering it with lotion several times a day. Not to mention I was suddenly struggling with my weight. I'd packed on ten pounds shortly after my fortieth birthday, for no apparent reason. Somehow, I swept these clear signs of perimenopause—and any related concerns about my fertility—to a far corner of my mind.

As I left my doctor's office, she handed me a lab slip and sent me home with instructions to get blood drawn on day three of my cycle, to test my FSH levels. I still wasn't ready to have a baby alone, but I was beginning to take action to get informed. This is exactly what I coached my clients to do when faced with a major decision—gather information and notice your reaction to it. At each step along the way, I'd either gather momentum to keep moving forward or I'd watch my motivation wane, indicating what I really wanted.

they said it couldn't happen

The blood test fell on a day in early June. I left shortly thereafter to attend a Tibetan Nyung Nay retreat in the Zuni Mountains in New Mexico, a three-day retreat for Chenrezig, the Buddha of Compassion, known to be extremely powerful for healing illnesses, purifying negative karma, and opening the heart for compassion. Doing even one Nyung Nay retreat is said to be equal to doing any other purification practice for three months. I was intrigued, on behalf of my own healing and in the interest of deepening my work as a coach and teacher.

The Qigong practice, as I was learning it, helped open the central channel, which is the main energetic meridian in the body, running straight through the vertical center of the body from the head to the perineum. Opening the central channel is a primary focus of my spiritual and healing systems, in part because it gives access to more heavenly or spiritual information and indeed in my experience this opening made me receptive to different spiritual information and ideas. During practice, once I was able to harmonize the body and open the central channel, my thoughts and perceptions started to change and that in turn shifted my beliefs. For example, one day in practice it felt like my entire body disappeared and I observed myself breathing in and out with what I perceived to be the entire universe. I was part of huge sheet that breathed in and out together, one integral part of an entire whole, connected to everything. This realization shifted my sense of myself as a separate being, fighting alone for what I wanted. This experience changed my orientation and beliefs. Other times when practicing Qigong, I continually bumped into a benevolent force so loving and beautiful that encountering it would bring me to my knees, crying tears of relief. Over time, I began to interpret that force as the divine. After bumping into it repeatedly, I eventually trusted in its continual existence, and I felt sure of the support it offered me. I developed faith in this support through my direct experience, not by being told what to believe. Though, at times, I was prone to forgetting to trust in that support.

Although Chris knew that a student would likely begin to bump into these different ways of seeing the world, which could be called spiritual beliefs, he never pushed a specific philosophy onto his students. Rather, he taught in a way to help his students recognize and make sense of their own experiences, claiming those experiences as their own. If students wanted more guidance about various spiritual beliefs, Chris encouraged those students to seek out spiritual masters to see whether their teachings resonated. He supported his students in sampling many different masters and traditions, to understand what they offered and how they differed. The teacher leading the workshop in the Zuni Mountains was a high-ranking Tibetan monk with whom Chris had been friends and to whom he had given healing treatments. Though Chris had attended many of his retreats, he would not be attending this one. I had joined a few fellow Qigong students in registering for the retreat, intent on expanding my learning.

I flew into Albuquerque and rented a car to drive to the retreat center. Around five o'clock that afternoon, with just three miles to go to the retreat center, my cell phone rang. I was navigating a deeply rutted red clay road, so I didn't pick up the phone. Once I made it past the gates of the retreat center, I paused to listen to the message. "We got your test results," said a matter-of-fact voice I didn't recognize. "Your FSH numbers are higher than we expected," she said. "Call us if you want to deal with your infertility."

I felt the ground fall away as a panic washed over me. Who was this person on the phone? Was she even qualified to call me with this news? There must have been some nuance she missed. Infertility was defined as trying to get pregnant for one year without success. Since I hadn't even started trying to get pregnant, the "infertility" label couldn't properly be applied to me, could it? *She should not have used the term "infertility" so brazenly,* I thought, as reality seeped in. My age, my numbers, my irregular cycle—no matter what term she used, I would face a steep climb if I decided I wanted a baby.

I couldn't sit still with these thoughts. I chose not to call the doctor for clarification. Instead, I pushed the message out of my mind and kept driving up the road to meet the retreat participants. If I kept going through the motions, I might not fall apart.

As soon as I stepped out of my car, I was enveloped by unbearably hot, dry winds. Thick smoke hung in the air from a nearby forest fire, making it impossible to see trees even a short distance away. Dread blanketed me like that smoke. Why in the world had I decided to attend this retreat? A two-day vow of silence? Thirty-six hours of fasting? What once sounded like a powerful cleansing ritual looked gruesome now.

For the next three days, I was packed sardine-style into a small stupa, with zero personal space. My knees touched students on either side of me, and I could feel the prayer book of the person behind me resting on my back. I plodded through the thick book of prayers, some of which were pages and pages long, repeating them fifteen times each. Where was the healing in *this*? In theory, mantra practice like this occupies the part of the mind that is constantly chattering, but it had no such effect on me. I spent three days with my body squished in an overcrowded stupa and my mind hooked by the message from the doctor's office. My own mantra supplanted the prayer book, repeating obsessively: *I want a baby,* while tears streamed down my face. Then all of a sudden I'd flip, marveling in the freedom of a childless life. Then I'd flip again, spiraling down a hole of self-pity, feeling betrayed that the prospect of motherhood may have been stripped from me. I didn't know for sure if I wanted a baby, but I did know that I wanted the decision to be mine—not my body's—to make. With evidence that my fertility door was rapidly closing, did I want to do the work to pry it back open?

∾

As soon as I had returned home from New Mexico, I made two phone calls. First, I called my doctor's office, relaying to the receptionist the very disturbing message about my supposed infertility.

"Oh, my, I'm so sorry," she exclaimed. "There's no way she said that."

I took a deep breath to settle my nerves. I decided not to debate the assistant's wording, focusing instead on what the message should have said. "Do you know what my FSH levels were?"

The receptionist transferred me to a nurse, who pulled up my file. "Your FSH was 23.5," she said. "It's quite high. I think that's why the message must have been left for you."

"Okay, thanks," I replied sourly. At the time, I didn't realize this number meant I was basically perimenopausal, and that having a child on my own was nearly impossible. Nor did I ask any questions about what the number meant. For now, I needed to believe that it was still medically possible to have my own baby. So I hung up the phone, thinking my numbers indicated I was facing an uphill battle toward pregnancy. I didn't know the half of it.

Then I called Chris to set up an emergency session. I needed to discuss this latest development with him. He said I could come over right away, and I took him up on it, jumping in my car for the short trip to his home in Albany, only fifteen minutes from my house. By the time I arrived, he had the table set up in his new treatment space, a little building in the back of his home.

Chris summoned me to one of the chairs he'd set up and asked me to sit down. Once we were facing each other, he began, "So, what's up? How can I help you today?" I noticed the note of caution in his voice, and I willed myself to remain calm.

I nodded so that he knew I had heard his question, but realized I could not speak. My neck and throat started contracting, and that familiar lump lodged itself in my throat. I don't know why I was trying not to cry. Chris had seen me cry a thousand times. But it seemed no matter how comfortable I had become crying in front of him, there was always a moment before I let go.

"My hormone levels are really bad," I said, releasing a wave of sobs. "I'm not sure I will be able to get pregnant if I want to." My voice cracked and my chest heaved. As the weight of my possible infertility pressed into me. I gave Chris a garbled rundown of the information I had received. He reached for a box of Kleenex and offered it to me as I continued. "They can't say I'm infertile," I insisted, "since I haven't even started trying to get pregnant yet."

"Okay, so your chemistry is off," Chris said, his soft brown eyes taking me in gently. "We can take a look at that. And where are you at with your decision otherwise?" Chris wanted to keep me focused on what I wanted, not the potential obstacles in my way.

"I don't know," I said with a note of frustration in my voice. "I still feel totally stuck. And if this turns out to involve a lot of medical intervention, I don't think I can afford to get pregnant, let alone raise a child."

As I spoke, my eyes started to well up again. Thinking about money always stirred panic in me. Over the past several weeks, when I'd thought about having a baby, I felt myself cut off the inquiry. The question of babies barely could be heard above the panic about finances.

"I understand it's scary not to know what's coming financially, but I fear that you will never feel like you have enough money to have a baby. It seems to be the nature of money—no one ever feels like they have enough," Chris said.

"Uh, yeah, I guess," I responded dejectedly. I knew his words were true, but I couldn't take them in, not fully at least.

"You've had a shock from your doctor's message," Chris concluded. "Let's put you on the table and help you return to yourself. You are too upset right now."

As I lay down face up on the table, knees propped up on

pillows, he worked silently for several minutes, and I allowed my tears to fall. My racing thoughts started to slow down, and my breath, which had been erratic, eased into a smooth rhythm. With a calmer mind, I asked Chris, "Do you think it's impossible for me to get pregnant?"

"I have no way of knowing," he said, explaining that he sees the body so differently than Western medicine, that he couldn't speak to the significance of their tests. "We *do* know that you have a very refined and delicate nervous system, though. Any amount of stress throws off your chemistry and hormone levels. We can look at that when the time comes, if you decide you want to move forward having a baby."

A wave of relief washed over me. I had a similar view of the body, and I wanted to retain hope that I could still get pregnant. I left the session feeling hopeful and calm.

You'd think the information from the doctor's office would have propelled me into action, but I spent another six months ruminating. Ultimately, Chris was inviting me to focus on the more important question: Do I want a baby? He understood there were many paths to motherhood, and if I chose to become a mother, I would find a way. He also knew me well enough to understand that contemplating the potential complications of late-in-life conception—sperm donor, egg donor—would have distracted me from recognizing my most deeply held desire. At this point, it was important to keep the question simple: Did I want to be a mother or not? Instead of jumping on the baby train, I spent another six months on the platform, hemming and hawing. In hindsight, this seems absurd. I should have dropped everything and begun trying immediately. But while in the thick of it, the decision loomed so large that even the daunting test results did nothing to move me forward.

maybe a sperm donor isn't so bad

"We picked our sperm," my friend Katie exclaimed to group of women sitting around a long rectangular table at an upscale Mexican restaurant in the Mission District. Katie, a former roommate of mine, and her partner, a Panamanian woman named Nilka, were a constant source of inspiration for me, never more so than now. Katie, who grew up in the Midwest, was the quintessential "salt of the earth." She had light red hair, freckled skin, blue eyes, a jubilant smile, and buoyant energy, even when she was being worn thin by her corporate law job. Nilka was her physical opposite: she was black, with warm brown eyes, and hair styled in short twists. Nilka exuded warmth and compassion. My visits with these two always left me energized.

Though everyone at the table was dialed into this conversation, I'm guessing I was a bit more curious than others. It was now fall, several months since the doctor's call, and I still hadn't made any real progress in my decision. "How did you pick it?" I asked from across the table.

"Well, we wanted a Latin Black donor, since Nilka won't have a genetic link to the child. We also wanted him to be tall, spiritual, and a college grad," Katie paused and laughed.

I marveled at Katie's list of characteristics. I hadn't even considered how to pick a donor. The criteria struck me as both strange and practical.

"It turns out it's impossible to find any Black Latino donors," Katie said. "And there are also very few Black donors, so it got narrowed down very quickly."

Nilka reached over and placed her hand onto Katie's, gently adding, "One of the potential donors was six-foot-four and over two hundred and fifty pounds, so we ruled him out, fearing it might make for a difficult birth."

We all laughed. Though I imagined many women the same size as Katie had partnered with equally large men, I thought it was endearing that Nilka wanted to look out for Katie in this way. Nilka glanced lovingly at Katie. "The donor we picked jumped out at us because he practices the same style of Buddhism as us."

They both seemed so relaxed and straightforward about it. Their casual confidence about such an enormous decision shocked me. I assumed that if I ever picked a donor, I would obsess about each characteristic, second-guessing what was important or even relevant. But neither Katie nor Nilka expressed any hesitation or doubt. The process was not weird to them in any way; it was simply part of their path toward pregnancy.

"So, what's the deal with sperm banks?" I pressed. "How do you get access and whatnot?" In nearly every aspect of my life, I was quick to jump online to do a Google search to educate myself and be proactive. Though I often thought about typing "sperm bank" into the search engine, I'd always found a way to distract myself so I remained ignorant about the most basic aspects of picking a sperm donor. I had no idea if I could access a database online, or whether I needed to visit the sperm bank in person. Friends who knew I was contemplating using a sperm donor had offered to accompany me to the sperm bank, but I never took them up on it.

"It's really easy," Katie exclaimed. "It's all online. You just register and then can look at brief profiles. But usually you have to pay some money to see the actual pictures and more detailed profiles." Katie stopped, her expression changing from "casual conversation" to "wait a minute . . ." And then she asked, "Why? Are you thinking about getting pregnant?"

"Yes. Well, I haven't decided yet, but I'm thinking about doing it alone," I stammered. Some of the women at the table that night knew I'd been deliberating, but others were taken completely by surprise. I heard a collective gasp. "What? How exciting." I scrambled to divert the conversation back to Katie and Nilka, hoping somehow to get more answers without hijacking the whole conversation.

I was a bit shy to admit to my lesbian friends that I felt uncomfortable using a donor. I didn't want to insult them. Using a donor was a requirement for Katie and Nilka, not a choice. It was just something lesbian couples did. But my situation was different. When I thought about using a donor, I was flooded with shame, fear and a sense of failure. It seemed like everyone I knew could find a partner with whom to have a baby, except me. Having a baby on my own had somehow come to signify what I was always afraid to admit: I was flawed and unlovable. "You guys are so casual about it," I said. "I'd worry about his medical background and health and whether or not he's good looking and smart." I thought about how I scrutinized every guy I dated, holding them up to such high standards none of them could pass. "How in the world could I trust a complete stranger that I would never meet? What if he's lame?"

"I don't know," responded Katie with a laugh, "it's something we've always known we'd need to use to get pregnant, so it doesn't seem that weird, I guess." Katie's exuberance was contagious. What if I adopted her casual, happy stance? What if I refrained from getting caught up in details and worry? How could I let go of the troubling parts and just move forward like Katie and Nilka?

After dinner, we all stood on the sidewalk outside, saying our good-byes. I sought out Katie and Nilka. I wanted to soak up every ounce of their attitude and hear every gory detail of how they had chosen their donor.

"We have a password. You should borrow ours!" Nilka offered. "Come over and we'll go through profiles together. It's fun." Her excitement was contagious. Now that I'd been exposed to just how simple and straightforward picking a donor could be, I was ready to explore the topic for myself.

❧

A few weeks later, I fell in dance class and tweaked both my ankles and knees. They weren't full-blown sprains, but I couldn't get around very easily. I knew from experience that my body healed much more quickly if I stopped at the first sign of injury rather than trying to push through. So, I decided to stay in bed for the weekend to heal. With my knees propped up on a pillow and my laptop perched on them, I pulled up Google and cautiously typed "sperm donors." Links for several sperm banks popped onto my screen. I found one that allowed me to sift through profiles without a lengthy registration process or fees. They didn't provide pictures, but in addition to the donors' physical characteristics and medical history, the profiles included narratives written by the staff, based on interviews with the donors. And there were extensive personal essays written by the donors themselves, answering questions like how would you describe your personality, what are your interests and hobbies, what are your goals, and what talents do you have?

I entered some broad search terms: five-foot-ten and above, any eye color, any complexion. I hit return, and I held my breath as I waited for the results to pop up. First up, a man from Peru who spoke three languages, played the violin, painted, and was majoring in Computer Science at UC Berkeley. The staff person who interviewed him noted, "This is probably the most attractive donor we have ever had." My heart started to race. He sounded like my dream guy. I'd always been attracted to South American men, and I loved the idea of this well-rounded guy who had developed both his scientific and creative side. I mentally filed him under "definite possibility" and continued my search, finding donors who had an amazing mix of creativity and brains.

Their personal essays revealed them to be gentle, caring men, another huge priority to me as I thought about the traits I wanted to be passed down to a future child. I was starting to get excited about using a donor. These men seemed more promising than any of the men I had dated recently. I allowed myself to try to picture the men, imagining how their list of physical traits and characteristics would blend with my own genes. Critics and cynics may argue that for many choosing a sperm donor borders on eugenics, but it didn't feel like that to me. While using a sperm donor was no longer a deal breaker, the prospect of picking a list of desired characteristics, made giving up the dream of procreating with a romantic partner palatable. It was still a far cry from what I had dreamed about when I had envisioned motherhood throughout my life. There was still an incredible list of unknowns and the sadness of using a stranger to conceive rather than a man I'd grown to love. But, if I allowed myself to relax and have an open mind, this sperm donor thing could actually be kind of fun.

there are no
guarantees in life

With the sperm donor hurdle cleared, I began to envision life as a single mom. Most of my hobbies and lifestyle choices would be sacrificed to a baby. Worse yet, I knew I'd be raising a baby without any family support. My parents, who lived more than a five-hour drive away, were both approaching eighty. Even if they wanted to help, I knew it would be hard for them to contribute in any substantial way. And my sister, who lived in Santa Cruz, wasn't crazy about babies. She'd never had her own children, and I couldn't envision her offering to babysit. This notion produced melodramatic visions of me completely isolated, never leaving the house again.

Once again, I sought Chris's counsel in a private session. As Chris began his treatment, I shared, "I've been thinking about how alone I will be raising a baby." I stammered bitterly, "You know my family, they won't help."

"If I know one thing about you, it's that you know how to create community," Chris responded. "You will not be raising a baby alone."

True. Throughout my life, I'd been the one to organize weekends away, dinner parties, wine tasting clubs, and more. I was constantly bringing friends from different groups together, building bridges and connections. I appreciated that Chris acknowledged this, but dinner parties and wine tasting clubs were one thing. Would that community spirit translate to raising a baby?

"And, there are no rules in this area," Chris coaxed. "You can pave your own path, create your own family, however you want that to look."

True again. There were no rules for the path I might undertake, but there was also no manual. I would be operating outside the realm of convention. I could define family however I wanted. I could invite friends to be aunties and uncles, even grandparents. I opened my mind to other unconventional ideas. I owned a big house, which was calling out for more people to live in it. I could offer an au pair or a college student free rent in exchange for help. I could even invite another single mother into the house as a roommate, and we could share the cost of an au pair. We might even be able to enter into a more formal co-parenting situation. Yes, I could construct whatever I wanted. There were no limits.

But even as my mind started to expand, the old message came back: I'd be single forever if I had a baby alone. "I feel like I'm making a choice between being in a partnership and having a baby. I just can't get over that fear of being alone."

"This is where you are confused," Chris chuckled. "There are never any guarantees in life. And certainly, that's more true with men," he joked. "Even if you get married and decide to have children together, there is no guarantee that he will stick around. He could leave you while you are pregnant or the day your baby is born. You have no idea what might happen. And conversely, you could get pregnant tomorrow and then meet the man of your dreams before you have the baby."

Chris was touching on one of the central teachings of Buddhism, impermanence; the notion that everything is transitory and changing and thus unpredictable. I'd been studying with a Thai monk named Luang Por Jamnian for several years. He'd hammered this point home, recounting a story about the Buddha, who had instructed students to sit in the charnel grounds, an aboveground site for the putrefaction of bodies, to watch the bodies decompose. By doing so, the student may eventually penetrate the idea that everything is impermanent. Luang Por Jamnian would do the same for us students, providing gruesome details of the charnel grounds, hoping we too might penetrate the notion of impermanence. For me, it had remained a concept. I understood it intellectually, but clearly it hadn't sunk in yet.

But now, as Chris was pointing at the ridiculousness of my thinking, the teaching was worming its way into my brain. It was such an obvious and yet profound epiphany. Because nothing in life is permanent or certain, I could not guarantee anything. It was impossible to predict which path to motherhood might leave me single or partnered, or how long I'd remain in any given state. As Chris continued to work on me, I settled down more and more, my mind opening. Attraction, too, must be completely unpredictable. It was ridiculous to assume no man would be attracted to me if I had a child. Who knew? If I already had my own child, that might eliminate the hot-button issue from my dating life. Men could come into my life, but they didn't need to father a child.

"I normally wouldn't do this," Chris said, "but you and I are close friends as well as student and teacher, and you are running out of time, so here it is. Every time you speak about not being able to have a baby, you burst into tears." He paused as if to allow me to take in what he was saying. "And, when you talk about having a baby, your nervous system calms down. I just want to reflect back to you what I see." Again he paused to let me take this in. I was ready to contradict him, but instead I allowed myself to try on his theory. "It's true that you can find a million reasons not to have a baby, but think with your heart, not your mind," he advised.

Really? Did I cry every time I talked about not being able to have a baby? In my mind, I was a basket case every time I talked about any aspect of the baby idea. But as I let his insight wash over me, the trend he'd been witnessing became clear.

Toward the end of the session, Chris said, "Get really quiet. Settle down and calm your system so you can hear yourself. Avoid the temptation to be busy all the time." I took in a deep breath as his words and touch quieted my system. I could tell that he was leading me to a very calm and settled place so that I could reference it later. "Let your true nature decide, not your fears and logic."

Ironically, this was the exact advice I'd always give my clients and friends, and it was a major tenant of Chris's teaching. I knew that when the mind was busy worrying about details and life, it remained in a state of constant chattering, obscuring the deeper wisdom. Usually I could notice and calm this in myself, but around the baby topic, I needed help.

"But I live such an easy lifestyle. I am settled down," I retorted. And of course, in comparison to where I had been several years prior when I left corporate law completely burnt out, I *was* settled down. In fact, if I compared myself to the vast majority of driven Bay Area friends, I looked like a Zen monk. Yet, if I were honest with myself, I would have seen that in the months I had been contemplating motherhood, I also was coming up with an endless number ways to keep myself in constant motion—a DIY project, a trip somewhere, a new business angle. It was my nature to get things done, to make things happen. So that's what I did, with no recognition that all the while I was avoiding the opportunity to settle down and listen to my deepest, truest desire.

Clarity was on its way, however slowly. I'd gotten over my fear of using a sperm donor; accepted the uncertain nature of life and partnerships; and decided that dating under the extreme pressure to procreate was a dead-end street, while dating after having a baby could be liberating. I could see interesting and exciting ways that I might construct the support and structure I would need to raise a baby and take care of myself financially. Though fears continued to surface, looping around in my brain, they had less power each time. I could see that having a baby alone would be hard, but it might actually be feasible. Now I had to decide once and for all: Do I really want to do this?

The answer would come in late January, during one of Chris's weekly Qigong classes. As Chris instructed us through the basic prostration exercise, we moved our hands around our bodies in a flowing pattern, down the back side of the body, up the front side, splitting in two at the heart center, and again down the back side of the body. "As you move your hands around the body, imagine that the hands are X-raying the body or combing through the body, sensing the quality of each part as you pass through it," Chris instructed. I knew the pattern well. It was the foundation for this style of practice. The objective was to split the body into the "hard side" and "soft side," or to separate in the mind's eye the supportive structure of the skeleton, from the soft, insubstantial, lively quality of the front side of the body. This exercise can also be understood as dividing the yin from the yang. The theory is that the *Qi*, or life force, and the *Shen* get dispersed by the stress of life. By separating the supportive structure from the receptive structure, the *Qi* becomes organized and contained, no longer dispersed. This invites the *Shen* of the body to return.

As we practiced that evening, I felt my body harmonizing. I no longer sensed the body as various parts—no shoulder joints or hip joints. I was becoming one continuous flow. To help the practitioner, instructors often use the image of the turtle and snake, and now as I practiced, this imagery was lighting up. The entire backside of my body was becoming an arc of shell, while the front was becoming hundreds of luminous snakes dancing. My perception of my body, which had now completely disappeared, morphed into the image of turtle and snake. I felt euphoric and calm at the same time.

After about an hour of class, we transitioned to sitting in chairs. Chris gave the familiar directions to sit at the edge of the chair so that our legs were bent at ninety-degree angles, supporting our backs. "Let the low back round slightly, without collapsing the upper body, while allowing the weight to drop squarely through the sit bones and into the legs," Chris guided. "Notice when you begin to lift away from the support of the ground by arching the back and slowly come back." Once we settled into this posture, he instructed us to reestablish our awareness of the hard side and soft side of the body, while also paying attention to the breathing. "Try to pay attention to the breathing without concocting it in any way. Just notice it as it is," he advised. With each in breath, I felt as if my being was immense, expanding in all directions. With each out breath, I felt my being melt deeper and deeper into this otherworldly state in which I had no body. It was as if my whole body was expanding and contracting with the universe in a beautiful union akin to prayer. In the deepest part of my being, I perceived a thin line of glorious light glowing within a perfectly clear shell. I recognized this as the *Shen*, or light, residing deeply in the body. This state welcomes wisdom and clarity, because one's essence or nature has returned home to the body.

Sure enough, as I was luxuriating in the expansion and contraction of my body, a vision came to me: a young baby girl dressed in bright pink on a swing. She was surrounded by a green, grassy field, which provided a beautiful contrast to her pink dress. She smiled and laughed as I pushed her on the swing. It was an easy moment of joy between the baby and me. And suddenly, just like that, my mind was made up. I wanted a baby. The reasons not to simply vanished. The years of indecision melted away. In that moment, the truth was so obvious, so clear that I was jolted by the idea that I ever could have thought that I didn't want a baby.

When the meditation ended, I came back to a normal mind and body, though that image of the baby girl on the swing remained. I sat with a sweet smile on my face, recalling the joy. I could tell that, with my normal mind, my head would still say no if I asked. But my heart knew the answer, and it was unwavering in its certainty.

As soon as class ended, I bounded up to Chris to share my epiphany. I could barely contain myself from doing a dance and leaping in the air with joy as I waited my turn to chat with him. "I figured it out!" I said gleefully. "I want a baby!"

"That's fantastic," he said, joining my enthusiasm. "Good job."

"Good job?" I asked, puzzled though not surprised, since it was not an uncommon answer for Chris.

"Yes, good job! By the sounds of it, you have finally stabilized in your knowing." Chris explained that as we had worked together through my year of debate, he had kept placing me in my clear mind of wisdom, in hopes that I would eventually stabilize there. "You had all these ideas that upset you and destabilized you about having a baby. They were so distressing to you that you would pop out of your knowing that you wanted a baby. I helped you clear away the impediments and misperceptions, so they couldn't distract you as much, until you finally came to understand what you truly wanted."

When I think back to this night, I still can't believe how deeply I had repressed my desire for a baby. Perhaps because we have more options today where motherhood is concerned, finding the right path can feel even more difficult. I had been striving to answer the baby question with the same mind that I bring to daily life—the logical, figuring-it-out-and-getting-things-done mind. But I couldn't access my wisdom from that place, because my chattering mind and worries about logistics kept me in a state of confusion. In Buddhism, there's a distinction drawn between the heart mind, or *jitta*, and the pure knowing, or *yana*. The heart mind is tied up with all worldly concerns, past life information, and other confusions. The pure knowing resides in the third eye and is devoid of confusion. It is the seat of wisdom. A realized being is thought to be able to reside continually in the pure knowing and is no longer disturbed by the heart mind. So yes, this former corporate lawyer living in the Bay Area's success-driven environment had a long way to go before she became fully realized. But I was practicing. When able to quiet the heart mind, I could rest in my pure knowing, allowing clarity to arise. And that clarity brought me right back home to my maternal longings.

"What were you like as a kid?" Chris had asked me once. "What did you think about and do?" An inquiry like this, he'd explained, could connect me to who I was before I'd become identified with ambition, before I'd begun worrying about pleasing my parents and others around me.

What was I like as a kid? I was a mama in the making, a baby-hungry child. Now, reunited with my true longing, I felt steadfast in my decision, ready to clear any obstacle that dared stand between my baby-to-be and me.

part 2: struggling

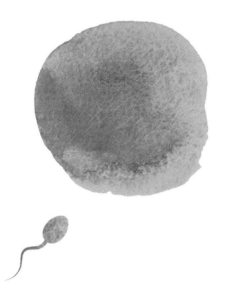

the hard truth

The next morning, I woke up ready to start getting pregnant, an enthusiasm tempered only by the nagging memory of that phone call from my gynecologist. "Call us if you want to deal with your infertility." Ugh. Armed with my new resolve, I scheduled an appointment and arrived eager to kick off Project Baby. "I'm ready to use a sperm donor and have a baby alone," I told my doctor.

"That's great," she said glancing down at my chart. "With your numbers, however, you should consult a reproductive endocrinologist immediately. It's very likely they'll tell you that you need to use an egg donor to conceive."

Those words knocked the breath out of me. My entire nervous system lurched forward and hung in suspense. I knew my FSH was bad, but bad enough to need an egg donor? "I understand my FSH isn't good," I said, more a question than a statement. I hadn't done any follow-up research on FSH; I had just accepted that it was high. The reality of that word "infertility" was starting to sink in. I had assumed the woman who had left that phone message had been mistaken or exaggerating. I further assumed that modern technology would help me overcome my issues. But an egg donor? I'd never once contemplated it. I'd heard about an acquaintance in college who had donated her eggs, but other than that I had no exposure to the idea. If sperm donation had initially seemed foreign to me, egg donation lived on another planet.

"That's true. Your Follicle Stimulating Hormone is 23.5," she responded, explaining that FSH gives an indication of how hard your body is working to ovulate. A high number means your body is working overtime, generating lots of FSH, just to produce one measly little egg, which doesn't speak well of the quality and quantity of your eggs.

A "good" number, she told me, is below nine. My number a few years earlier, when I'd taken preliminary tests to see how my fertility was looking, was eight. Though my doctor had cautioned me the number *could* change radically at any time, I'd brushed it off. Now the sharp spike to 23.5 shocked me.

I wasn't ready to go straight to a reproductive endocrinologist or fertility doctor to explore IVF, and I certainly was not going to entertain an egg donor at this point. I wanted to conceive as naturally as possible, and I wanted to have a baby genetically related to me. If I had to use an egg donor, I didn't think I wanted to get pregnant. Apparently my firm decision that yes, I wanted to be a mom more than anything, was laden with several contingencies.

Despite my doctor's strong recommendations, I was looking for other options. "I don't want to do IVF," I confessed.

"You could also do intra-uterine inseminations, or IUIs, here at the doctor's office or with a home midwife," she told me. She explained that an IUI used a catheter to inject "washed sperm" through the cervix and directly into the uterus. The sperm is "washed" to remove the seminal fluid which does not enter the uterus in traditional intercourse. "But again," she said, "I wouldn't recommend it. The odds would be minimal. But I understand that you need to do whatever is necessary to get closure before moving on to donor eggs."

I shuddered at her words, completely rejecting the notion of an egg donor. I had put up a barrier, and every time she suggested egg donation, I held up that barrier, deflecting the words before they could penetrate my psyche. I wasn't going to be getting closure before moving to egg donor. I was going to get pregnant on my own, or likely give up on the dream of having a baby.

"But it only takes one egg, right?" I asked incredulously. She had said "odds," hadn't she? And didn't odds imply possibility?

"Well, yes. But as you age the quality and quantity of your eggs decrease significantly. Miracles do happen. But I'd give you less than one percent chance of conceiving. Then again, it's true that someone is that one percent. I'm not going to tell you it's impossible, but it is improbable."

I peppered her with more questions about logistics, insurance coverage, and costs before I headed home for an intense make-out session with my research buddy, Google.

On my drive home, even though I was trying my hardest to ignore my doctor's blunt suggestion to use an egg donor, my mind was obsessing. My whole life, I'd been fascinated by the nature verses nurture debate. Part of what I was excited about when it came to having a child was the question of how my traits might express in my baby. I was doubly interested in this now, since I wasn't going into this with a partner who would have a genetic connection to the baby. If neither a partner nor I had a genetic link to the baby, wouldn't that be like adopting a child? Though I know many people who have had rich and fulfilling experiences with adoption, I had never contemplated that path toward parenthood, so the parallel didn't help me feel any more ready to use an egg donor.

In the same week that I emerged with unwavering conviction about having a child, I was informed that I'd likely need both an egg and a sperm donor to get pregnant. My whole body wilted with sadness.

Once home, my logical mind, determined to fight this perceived injustice, sprung into gear. A new mantra filled my mind, "You need only one good egg." I believed the only fulfilling way to have a baby was to use my own eggs, so my lawyer brain locked on a singular goal: figure out how to beat the odds.

Nestled in a comfy leather chair in my living room, I Googled "high FSH." Fertility clinic websites laid out the cold, hard facts. An FSH level above twenty is considered by some doctors to be consistent with perimenopause or premature ovarian failure. My high FSH, coupled with my age, gave me a 1-4 percent chance of conceiving. Even with all the fertility and assisted conception technology, research suggested nothing medical could be done to improve FSH levels. Again and again, the websites offered one solution to my problem: egg donation. Clearly a reproductive endocrinologist would either tell me it was impossible to get pregnant with my own eggs, or, best-case scenario, attempt to convince me to try IVF. I wasn't willing to fill my body with hormones and drugs in a last-ditch attempt to get pregnant, so to me the best-case scenario was a no-case scenario.

I decided I needed a sounding board, so I called my friend Annette, an older woman whom I often referred to as my surrogate mother, though really the correct term would probably be adopted mother. I met her through my coaching school, in a business support group, when we were first getting our coaching practices off the ground. Despite our age difference, we bonded instantly. She was the quintessential hippie woman, with a bold, wise spirit. She had two sons my age. She was a mentor and sounding board for me, always listening without judgment and giving it back to me straight, while showering me with immense love and dedication. In other words, she was the kind of mother I had always dreamed of having.

Annette knew I'd been contemplating single motherhood. She'd been around and around with me as I debated what to do, but I had not yet told her that I had made the decision once and for all. She picked up her phone with her regular cheery tone, "Hello, my sweet Sarah, how are you?"

"I'm pretty good," I responded. I cut to the chase with my news. "I finally decided that I am going to try to have a baby alone."

"Yeah, I'm going to be a grandma again!" she rejoiced. I could feel her enthusiasm as she launched into a stream of eager questions that I had to cut off before she got too excited.

"Annette," I said, "the doctor has told me that I have a very small chance of being able to conceive." I filled her in on the details. "A fertility doctor would be able to offer me some more testing that would potentially paint a clearer picture of my fertility. But, I'm worried that more tests will just paint a dismal picture, and I don't want to quash my lasts reserves of hope around getting pregnant." Having been a Feldenkrais practitioner and healer for many years,

I had seen many instances in which a negative diagnosis robbed a person of the power to change their body for the better. People easily rigidify around their diagnosis. It becomes their mantra, an obstacle rooted in their path, immovable and unchangeable. As a result, they lose their ability to create positive change even when the possibility is present. To avoid locking up on possibility, I needed to preserve my hope and faith. As far as I could tell, having more numbers and diagnoses was not going to help me in this arena.

"Do you think I'm crazy to skip the fertility doctors for now and try to beat the odds on my own?" I asked. "I've already been researching natural fertility enhancement and found tons of women who lowered their FSH and improved their egg quality with herbs, lifestyle adjustments, meditation, and things like acupuncture, or naturopathy."

"Oh, sweetie, I think you should do whatever your gut tells you is right and whatever allows you to move forward without regret," she said, her loving reassurance pouring through the phone.

My research had confirmed what I already believed—that alternative and complementary medicine took a different view of fertility. For one, they saw fertility as part of a larger whole. So improving the function of the entire system could support the reproductive system to operate optimally, balancing hormones and reducing stress, which negatively impacts the reproductive system. In terms of fertility, Chinese medicine, including acupuncture and Qigong, does not believe that a woman's body has a finite number of eggs that age and die in a woman's late thirties and early forties. These disciplines believe that our access to the eggs slows down, almost like the reproductive system goes to sleep. "With proper diet, nutrition, balance and energetic practice, it's believed that women can revive their egg reserve, and wake up the reproductive system. There are even some modern medical studies that support this notion of the reproductive system," I shared, hope returning as I spoke.

"Well, I know that you are *very* in touch with and connected to your body. And when you set your mind to something, you get it done." We both laughed at that understatement about my obvious, bullheaded tenacity. "And you have so many resources for healers in Chris and beyond. I think it's reasonable to give it a shot."

"Thank you," I said tearfully. In the glow of Annette's reassurance, I could feel my truth emerge. I needed to do this. I had to make the effort. What other choice did I have, when for me using an egg donor was most definitely not an option?

To someone unfamiliar with alternative medicines, my belief that I could improve my fertility naturally could seem completely insane. But this was my world. I'd been interested in alternative and complementary medicine since college. I firmly believed (and still do) that there are legitimate, alternate ways to view the body and its health. Allopathic, or Western medicine as it's often called, is simply one paradigm for health, which focuses on germs and pathogens. Chinese medicine, another time-tested paradigm, focuses on balancing the organs and the *Qi*, or the life force. Ayurvedic medicine, meanwhile, sees the body as a balance of the various doshas, or physical and mental constitutions.

Through my work with Chris, I'd experienced firsthand a completely different view of the body. Many times when I brought an ailment to Chris, I would start off with a description of what was going on in my body from a Western point of view. He would stop me and say, "I don't see the body the same way, so I can't comment." Yet through his particular style of bodywork and healing, he had cured my body of several illnesses and mysterious ailments. For instance, when I'd begun developing superficial blood clots in my legs, I went for a full work up with Western doctors, including several specialists in various fields. But the cause of my clots remained a mystery. Then I had a session with Chris, to see if he could address the clots. "I can see exactly why they are happening," Chris said. "The *Qi* in your legs is very dispersed and disorganized." He did one session, and I've never had another clot again.

The world in which I lived was full of astounding healing stories that defied my notions of possibility. I'd even met a woman who'd been diagnosed with advanced breast cancer, who refused to seek traditional Western treatment. Instead she received treatments solely from Qigong master Zhixing. Within a year, her cancer was in remission. In this context, attempting to beat nine-ty-nine-to-one odds, in the service of my dream of genetic motherhood—well, it didn't seem strange at all. In fact, it seemed the only way to go.

After hanging up with Annette, I hesitantly called Chris. He was so generous with his time, and he was always available to talk to me. I didn't want to take advantage of his generosity, since he rarely charged for time on the phone. But I was weary from a long day spent in doctor's offices and Internet searches and overall anxiety, and this issue felt urgent to me.

When I reached him, I wasted no time giving him the rundown of the situation. "What do you think I should do?"

"Well," Chris considered, "I definitely think you are right that having a poor diagnosis from a fertility doctor is not going to help you. I think getting pregnant is one-part about fertility and another part about the inexplicable. It's mysterious what causes a life to form. But the importance of believing it's possible can't be understated."

I nodded along, as if he could see me.

"You need to do whatever will help you feel like you did your best. You have a lot of support out there. It's possible that grace may intercede and give you what you want." But Chris cautioned me to set some limits. "You need to have some measure of when you have done your best, so that you can move on. Set some criteria." He paused and took a breath. "Look, decide how much money you are willing to throw at the outside chance of beating the odds, and go for it. Stop when you reach that financial limit. But also decide how long you are willing to try. Decide if it's six months, a year, or whatever and don't go beyond that."

Chris's words rang true for me. I could already see that it would be very tempting to keep going, sinking tons of money into my dream of having a child with my own genetic material. There would always be the promise of one more theory or approach calling me to keep going. In hindsight, I realized this was a crucial piece of advice, and one that I would later incorporate into my own suggestions to women considering pregnancy. I learned, from my own efforts and supporting many other women on the journey, that it is easy to continue trying indefinitely, with no measure of when it's time to move on. It's easy to be lured by the hope of one last treatment unless you've set some limits ahead of time.

I wasn't sure I could delineate what it would look like to do my best. But time and money limits were clear to me, so I set them, fully believing, perhaps foolishly, if anyone could tackle the unfavorable odds, it was me.

The next morning, I woke up in make-it-happen mode. I scurried around setting appointments, starting with my naturopath who specialized in endocrinology. Then I set to work researching acupuncturists. I found a female Chinese acupuncturist, Dr. Lee, who had written a book (which I immediately ordered) and developed an entire protocol to improve fertility, helping many unlikely couples conceive against the odds. I made an appointment. After that, I read about various herbs and supplements to fortify the reproductive system. I cross-referenced the ones that made sense to me and ordered those. Then I began my Fertility Tour, visiting my various practitioners, who practiced all over the Bay Area.

First up was Dr. Lee, whose San Francisco office was plastered with pictures of happy families and notes thanking her for making their dreams come true. Would I someday send a picture of my own child to Dr. Lee? Upon arrival, I was greeted with a cup of "fertility tea." My treatment began with an intricate Chinese massage sequence designed to stimulate the relevant acupuncture points for fertility, performed by a man whose name I never learned. He then lit a match and warmed the air inside a series of small glass cups, which he set down on my oiled back and started moving in what felt like an elaborate, choreographed dance. At least one hour later, Dr. Lee finally appeared, her warm demeanor pervading the room. She checked my pulses and examined my tongue to assess where to place needles. Then she reviewed my history with me in great detail, asking seemingly endless questions about all aspects of my life. At the first possibility, I asked, "Do you think it's possible that I could improve my FSH and get pregnant?"

"Yes, of course," she said without hesitation. Her confidence gave me confidence.

After treating me with needles, Dr. Lee explained the entire regimen, which included rubbing my belly clockwise several times a day, ingesting several essential oil blends, and stimulating points related to reproduction by burning something called moxa, an herb formed into an incense-like stick, a few inches from important acupuncture points on my skin, a few times a day. As if that weren't odd enough, she also instructed me to buy a black-skinned chicken, something I'd never even seen before, let alone eaten, to make a bone broth every week, into which I would add Chinese herbs. Then came the supplements. The doctor's assistant lined up several bottles of pills and spent twenty minutes explaining which ones to take, how to mix the powders, and how to apply essential oils. There were completely different regimens for the first half of my menstrual cycle and the second half. I was going to need a personal assistant to help me get this all straight.

When I left Dr. Lee's office three hours later, I fought my way through the nearby Chinese market to buy the black-skinned chicken and other ingredients for the broth. What would my former law colleagues think of me now, elbowing my way out of the market with my chicken carcass, complete with head and feet, and bag full of mystery herbs? What would I say? Two words: *I'm desperate*.

As I drove home, back across San Francisco and the Bay Bridge, I felt the chicken magic working—I felt hopeful, uplifted. Dr. Lee, a fertility expert, did not think I was crazy for avoiding the endocrinologist and trying to beat the odds. She seemed just eccentric enough to have mysterious healing abilities beyond the technique of acupuncture.

I approached my fertility regimen dutifully, as if it were my full-time job. Five times a day, I sat down to the towers of pills and tinctures that took up a large piece of real estate in my small kitchen. I spent nearly fifteen minutes swallowing upwards of twenty pills at the end of each meal, after which I could hear water sloshing in my belly making me wish I hadn't eaten at all. But the repercussions of taking those pills on an empty stomach? No thank you. Next came the oils I rubbed on my belly, then the moxa burning, then my daily breathing and visualization exercises.

As if this weren't enough, I made the next stop on my Fertility Tour, back across the Bay Bridge to a different San Francisco neighborhood, Potrero Hill, to the office of my naturopath, Erica. Thin, blonde, and glowing with health, Erica had an approach to naturopathy that I loved. She looked at the synergy between various systems in the body, such as the hypothalamic–pituitary–adrenal axis (HPA axis or HTPA axis), which involves the balance between neurotransmitter levels, reproductive hormones, and stress hormones such as cortisol. She ordered various tests to evaluate the three interrelated systems in hopes of harmonizing them.

As we sat in her small but cozy office, I explained, "I want to get pregnant, but my FSH is really high. I'm hoping I might be able to change it and get pregnant naturally." As she looked over the labs I had brought from my OB/GYN and the tests she and I had completed over the past few years, I fidgeted nervously. When I couldn't stand the silence anymore, I added, "I keep thinking, I only need one egg."

"That is true," she said as she placed my paperwork back down on her desk. "I think it's possible to improve some things, which might help. And as you know, we need to address the whole system."

Before she could continue, I handed over the list of herbs I'd researched. "What do you think about these?"

She spent a moment looking them over before she replied. "Yep, these make sense," she said. "Chaste Tree is definitely helpful. It's nicknamed the 'women's herb' because it's used to treat premenstrual symptoms, menopause, and infertility." We went through the rest of the list, making a few tweaks and adding some others. Erica also recommended that I clean up my diet, eliminating sugar, alcohol, dairy, and gluten. I had read similar suggestions online, so I was ready to change my diet accordingly. Stop two on my Fertility Tour left me, once again, feeling validated and optimistic. No one seemed to think I was crazy to be trying.

Of course, Chris was stop three. I continued my sessions with him to help harmonize my body and support my health as much as possible. Over his years as a healing practitioner, he had noticed that as women age their pelvic regions experience more swelling and stagnation. So he focused on removing cold, stale energy—called *binqi*—from my pelvic region. Also, during times of stress, resources get shunted away from the non-crucial systems, so he helped me reduce my stress level, smoothing out my nervous system.

With these three powerful healers on my fertility team, I felt confident my plan was going to work.

The next step in Project Baby: I needed to learn everything I could about my cycle so I could time insemination perfectly.

Most women, and even doctors, rely on Ovulation Predictor Kits (OPKs) to determine the twenty-four to forty-eight-hour window before ovulation when luteinizing hormone (LH) spikes. A few days before suspected ovulation, you pee on these little sticks in hopes of detecting "the LH surge." These sticks, infamous to anyone who's tried to time ovulation, are considered the gold standard in predicting the release of the ovum from the ovary. But they were soon to become the bane of my existence. No matter how many sticks I peed on, I was not exhibiting a clear LH surge.

I took a step further, ordering *Taking Charge Of Your Fertility*—the bible for women who want to improve their chances of conception—aiming to become an expert in my cycle and all the signs and symptoms that went along with it.

The fertility bible taught me that the most important ovulation sign is the basal body temperature (BBT), the lowest body temperature attained during sleep. During the first half of a woman's cycle, estrogen dominance cools the body's temperature. As soon as she ovulates, progesterone dominates her system, which raises the body temperature by about half a degree or more. Therefore, tracking BBT indicates that ovulation has occurred. Tracking, however, can be a bit of a comedy, since you need to capture your temperature before you actually wake up and start moving, and you're required to record the temperature to the tenth of a degree. That's right, in a complete daze, half asleep and barely able to see, I was supposed to reach over to my bedside table to find the thermometer while moving minimally to avoid elevating my temperature and to remember to record the temperature rather than just thinking, *Never mind I'll remember it.* Of course I rarely recorded it in the moment, and regularly questioned whether I remembered it correctly hours later when I was ready to record the data. In fact, more than once, after my morning fog wore off, I couldn't remember if I'd taken my temperature, let alone the results.

After trying in vain to get accurate BBT records, I realized I could not be alone in this problem, so I scoured Amazon for a solution. Indeed, I found thermometers that save the last temperature for you. I still had to remember to *take* my temperature in the morning, but at least I wouldn't be responsible for charting the results before I was fully conscious. Despite my fancy new thermometer, I learned that while BBT indicates that ovulation has already occurred, the cervical fluid is actually what tells you when you are close to ovulating. And since insemination needs to happen before you ovulate, it's important to time it when it the cervical fluid is wet and slippery. The rise in BBT will then tell you whether or not you timed insemination properly. But my cervical fluid was so minimal it was hard to deduce anything from it. And my cycle so irregular that I could not deduce any patterns that might help me in future cycles.

Luckily, *Taking Charge of Your Fertility* enumerated several other signs and symptoms for tracking ovulation. For example, I bought a tiny microscope to analyze my saliva. Most days of the month, salvia just looks like a bunch of clumpy spots, but right before ovulation, estrogen spikes, causing saliva to form intricate patterns that look like little ferns. This blew my mind. Also, I began tracking my cervical fluid, which changes from thick and creamy to the thin, translucent consistency of egg whites at ovulation.

My original plan had been to track my cycle for a few months to learn its rhythms. Theoretically, armed with three months of tracking data, I'd be able to predict when I should inseminate.

By then it would be May, and I thought I might put my efforts on hold until after attending a Qigong retreat in England with Chris's Qigong master, Zhixing. I'd been to study with him twice before and was in awe of him and his teaching. I was dead set on not trying to get pregnant until after I attended that retreat, figuring that my chances of going after I had a baby were slim to none.

But after a month of meticulous, dedicated, albeit sometimes blurry-eyed research, none of my symptoms lined up—my BBT was all over the map, my cervical fluid revealed nothing, my saliva looked like . . . saliva, and my OPK sticks produced nothing near a positive result. I concluded unequivocally that my cycle was completely erratic, bordering on non-existent. I started to rethink my plan. I consulted Chris to ask his opinion about when I should start trying to conceive.

"I think time is running out," he cautioned. "I'd get on it as soon as possible. Zhixing isn't going anywhere. But your fertility is finite."

Giving up my dream of seeing Zhixing that summer wasn't going to be easy. And yet, I suspected Chris was right—my fertility was headed downhill. Still I gripped onto that dream with my mental claws and held tight. Looking back, I'm not sure if I simply hadn't made pregnancy priority one yet, or if I really didn't understand the gravity of the situation. Either way, I didn't view a few months' delay as material to my pregnancy attempts, though I know now that a few months can make a big difference for women exhibiting symptoms like mine.

After tracking that first cycle, I started again, tracking for a nail-biting fifty-three days before my temperature spiked, indicating that I'd ovulated. Every day I took my temperature, analyzed my saliva, tried to make sense of cervical fluid, and peed on OPK sticks. I continued to eat like a saint and consume copious supplements. I entered the data into various apps on my phone, but nothing about my cycle made any sense. At one time, I had noted the ferning pattern in my saliva but I never had a positive OPK or temperature spike. I had very little, if any, cervical fluid, so I couldn't detect any pattern there. What did it all mean for my fertility? The question frustrated and worried me, constantly. On Thursday, May 10, I finally got my period, which meant that my cycle had been sixty-seven days long. I'd never been so happy to get my period. And yet, I was disheartened by just how irregular my cycle had become. *I'd be stupid to run off to England rather than seizing this opportunity to inseminate.* If all went well, I would ovulate in ten to fourteen days. Finally, I got it: forget about Zhixing; I *had* to do an insemination that cycle.

Of course, this meant I could need the sperm samples within the next ten days. Since I'd originally planned to track for a few months to gain data, I had neither started picking out a sperm donor, nor considering options for insemination. I jumped into action.

spermland

Sperm shopping wouldn't be easy. This I knew. For one, I'm a little crazy when it comes to making decisions in general. I need to know *all* my options, and I need to consider each *exhaustively* before I make my choice. Options abound in Spermland, and, like a Christmas shopping countdown, my time was limited. For two, choosing half my child's genetics felt monumental to me, even more important than timing insemination. I enlisted Chris for help.

"Sure," he agreed after class one day. "Go through the profiles and narrow it down to about ten donors. Then I will go through them with you and help you decide."

Chris has an intuitive gift. By looking at a picture, hearing a person's voice, or any number of other means, he can sense the person's health. Knowing he'd back me up in this decision boosted my confidence. In that moment, I could feel my self-doubt coming to throw me off balance so I asked for more guidance. "How should I approach picking my top ten?" I asked, fidgeting and shifting my weight from side to side.

"You are more intuitive than you realize," Chris reminded me. "Calm your mind and tune into the profiles. You'll know. Certain donors will resonate with you and others will have a chemically repellant aspect. The donors that resonate will be sticky and more likely to get you pregnant. Look for that."

The next morning, I followed Chris's advice, engaging in Qigong meditation before opening my laptop to search profiles. I practiced until my mind stopped its incessant chatter and I could focus on my breathing and other bodily sensations. Once I felt grounded, I shifted over to my bed and revved up the computer.

The logical first step in picking out a sperm donor should have been choosing a sperm bank. Unlike most other medical services, sperm banks are ungoverned, meaning they make up their own policies and regulations, which vary widely from bank to bank. For instance, the banks' limits on the number of offspring one donor can produce range from ten to sixty. Their screening, tests, and criteria for donors differ significantly. Their rules for sperm purchase and use, the amounts and types of information they provide in donor profiles, their policies for donor contact, their practices for tracking how many live births a donor produces, their shipping abilities and policies—none of these are regulated. Considering my background in legal policy and medical ethics, it's remarkable that I didn't research or even question these details. I had tunnel vision, directed at one goal and one goal only: finding the right donor. I would choose the bank where I found the "right" donor, and I would make that decision based on the intuitive feeling I got from the donor profiles.

I started with three banks. The profiles included everything from medical histories, to personal essays, to staff feedback about the donors, to baby pictures. A few even included audio files.

While some people go donor shopping with a grocery list of desired characteristics, I had very few. My number one priority was to find an Open Identity Donor (or Identity Release Donor), meaning my child could contact their donor upon their eighteenth birthday. Everything I'd read suggested that, for a donor-conceived child, this option was significant. But again, I was ignorant about how much these programs varied between sperm banks. I've since learned that some banks check in with their donors regularly to make sure they have current contact information, while others leave it to the donors to update on their own. Some banks will actively facilitate contact, while other banks will simply provide a last-known contact. Since most donors are college-aged young men, relying on their ongoing self-reporting and trusting their willingness to welcome contact more than eighteen years after they donated seemed shaky at best. Unfortunately, I could choose an Open ID donor, thinking I was guaranteed contact for my future child, when in reality many donor-conceived young adults can't find their donors when they try.

The rest of my criteria fell into the "ideal but not 100 percent necessary" category. I wanted the donor to be five-foot-ten or taller, since I'm only five-two. Given my own logical, methodical, intellectual, research-till-you-can't-research-no-more tendencies, I figured I should try to balance my kid out with a little creative, artistic, or even impulsive spark. I wanted someone good-looking and confident (who doesn't?), but liked to see a sweetness or a softness blended in. I wasn't looking for the jock. Perhaps my years in the Bay Area left me partial to the sensitive metrosexual? Also, I'm fair-skinned, but I had always been a sucker for the proverbial Latin Lover, spending my vacations in Cuba, South America, Mexico, Italy, and Spain. So, of course I was attracted to that in a donor.

The longer I searched, the more flustered I became, as if each profile I opened released a thousand chirping questions into the room. With Chris's advice in mind, I tried to follow my intuition, but self-doubt crept in, making it virtually impossible to trust who I was drawn to or repelled by based on personal essays and baby pictures. Some of these donors barely wrote two sentences on the page, and yet could I really trust the more loquacious ones were telling the truth? And baby pictures—how could I read my attraction to them? I'm a dyed-in-the-wool baby-luster. To me, all babies are cute. As for the audio files that I thought would guide my intuition—well, some of them did. But one of the sperm banks that provided audio files was located on the East Coast, and this California girl's internal compass could not find north in those thick, unfamiliar accents.

After a few hours, I took a break to call Annette for a sanity check.

"For the most part, there are only baby pictures. It's so hard to tell anything about what the guys are like from a baby picture,"

I told her. "This whole process is like some weird form of online dating," I remarked, letting out a big sigh. The irony was almost too much to bear.

Annette laughed. "Oh jeez, that's hard. I can imagine how strange it is. So, how are you going to choose someone?"

"I don't know. The audio files are the most helpful. It immediately gives me a picture of their personality, confidence, and whether they are smart, nice, funny, or sincere."

"That makes sense," Annette said reassuringly.

"But, it's amazing how many guys are so flippant responding to the personal essay questions. They give one-word answers, and sometimes they try to be funny when the questions are pretty serious. Many of them admit they are donating because they need money. But other answers seem corny or shallow."

I wondered how many of these young men had thought about their answers from a recipient's point of view, or what it would be like for their offspring to read their profiles? Had those who lacked sincerity avoided thinking too deeply about the ramifications of becoming a donor? Regardless, I was keenly aware that I'd be showing my future child the profile of his donor, and I didn't want that file to include anything specifically off-putting.

Annette, however, found the whole thing funny, which helped ease my tension—exactly why I had called her in the first place. "Why do they respond flippantly?" she wondered aloud. "I thought it was difficult and competitive to become a sperm donor?"

"Me too," I sighed.

"Keep going, sweetie. Focus on what makes sense to you. So if you like the audio files, prioritize those. And Chris is right, you are very intuitive, so don't second-guess yourself."

After hanging up with Annette, I continued my search. Just speaking my thoughts to another person cleared the doubt from my brain. It was one thing to choose to become a single mother, but orchestrating the creation of another human alone? That was another thing entirely. I was going to need a sounding board and witness from time to time.

While I was culling through profiles, Chris was in the midst of remodeling a house he had recently bought in San Francisco and was traveling around the US teaching more than usual. So when I was ready for him to chime in, I sent him my passwords for the various sperm banks and we scheduled a phone session.

"So, how'd you do?" Chris asked when I called. I sheepishly told him that even though he had told me to narrow it down to about ten donors, I had a much longer list, probably about twenty or so, spread across the three sperm banks.

We began with one of my favorites, the well-rounded, attractive Peruvian man, who had initially caught my attention when I first looked at sperm donors. But Chris axed him, declaring, "I get an immediate 'no.'" I can't even read more than two sentences of his profile because he is so strange. The reason he wants to be a sperm donor is very odd. It's like he wants to propagate the world with his semen because he thinks so highly of himself."

Over the next hour and a half, we shaved my pile down, eliminating donors based on reported health histories, essay answers, my firmly-held desire for an Open ID donor, and Chris's intuitive takes on their overall wellness. At last two remained: a Turkish guy and someone we referred to as the "all-around nice guy," whom we both liked. The Turkish guy was in grad school, seemed incredibly smart, spoke two languages, played an instrument, and had the dark features I yearned for. The all-around nice guy captained his volleyball team, studied mechanical engineering, spoke French, and played the piano. He seemed straightforward, uncomplicated, and well-liked by the staff members who had commented on him, and his coloring matched mine: blondish brown hair and light eyes.

"This seems like one of the most important decisions I've ever made in my entire life," I told Chris. "Do you mind talking through these last two?"

"Sure," Chris said patiently. "I definitely like the Turkish guy. He's very interesting. On paper, he's not really a match. But from a more esoteric view, he's really great. It's hard to explain, but there is something about him. It's a good match."

"I know," I said. "He just looks so dorky." He'd been a very cute kid, yet his baby pictures were unusual. Possibly because they were taken in Turkey, they had a different quality to them. The little boy in the image was dressed in what I would characterize as a bad JC Penny outfit from the '70s, with suspenders and knee socks. In another picture he wore a comical little beanie hat.

This typifies what donor selection is like: the decision feels enormous, but the information provided is so sparse that tiny details like the clothes and pictures take on extraordinary weight. Maybe it's a testament to how strange the donor selection process can be. I found myself latching onto small details to extrapolate into the donor's overall character, or grasping at other details to help make one donor stand out over the others. Obscuring his identity further, the Turkish donor's written profile was short and curt. He was undoubtedly smart, and I loved that he spoke two languages and played an instrument. I've always been attracted to foreign men and different cultures, so he intrigued me. Yet I imagined showing my child his profile and having to explain that, although his photo was not flattering and he wrote very little, on some other level, he was the right guy.

When I confessed that I was having trouble connecting to the answers in his profile and his pictures, Chris didn't flinch. "I understand," he said. "But he's healthy and very sticky."

Then we turned to the all-around nice guy. With him, I got hung up on his audio file. When the interviewer asked which holiday he liked best, he explained that he liked Thanksgiving more than Christmas, because he didn't think Christmas was as much fun as an adult, when he had to start buying presents for other people and didn't receive as many presents in return. However, this childish answer was balanced by his enthusiasm for a 3,800-mile bike ride he made across the US, which he described as the most important decision of his life.

I told Chris about the Christmas comment. "I would hate for my child to hear this." I realized I was grasping, but I couldn't help myself. With such a dearth of information, each little detail took on such incredible significance.

"I don't think anyone is going to be perfect," Chris said. "He's young. Don't get too caught up on the details."

"Ahhh, I don't know!" I exclaimed in frustration. "Okay, thanks for your help. I'll mull these over and figure it out."

"Sarah," Chris caught me just before I hung up, "don't forget that genes probably only account for a small percentage of how a child turns out. The intrinsic character of the child is responsible for so much, and how that works remains a mystery. Then you add upbringing into the mix and the actual genetic code fades further yet into the background. So don't get too hung up on this process. Trust that you will make the right decision."

If by "don't get too hung up" Chris meant "don't carry your computer around for the next few days, whipping it out to ask friends' opinions on these profiles any chance you get," then I suppose I allowed myself to get a little too hung up. I accosted my roommate Armene one afternoon while she was trying to cook herself dinner. I plopped my computer down on the kitchen counter next to her cutting board and started rattling off details about each donor, flipping back and forth between the pictures of each. "But wait," I said, "you have to hear what he says about Christmas in his audio file and tell me what you think. Is it too ridiculous?"

"No, it's kind of endearing," she said. "But I understand why it bothers you when you have so little other information about him." I continued on, bombarding her with every last detail.

And so it went, quizzing my friends, tossing and turning at night, continually envisioning what my baby would look like and act like with the two different donors. I read their profiles obsessively, opening my computer over and over to see their pictures afresh. I even took screen shots, so I could look at the donor pictures side by side. But I still couldn't choose, and I was running out of time.

I revisited Chris's idea of "stickiness" many times, trying to imagine which of these two donors I would have been more likely to date or simply to gravitate toward if I saw him at a party. But that was impossible—not to mention creepy—since I had only baby pictures.

Two days later, after spending so much time considering, my intuition made a clear connection: I would use the all-around nice guy. As soon as I made the decision, the choice seemed obvious, as if he had been the only right answer all along. In the end, I just didn't feel enough synergy with the Turkish guy. The all-around nice guy, was just that—well rounded and liked by everyone. That had to be worth something.

Taking this huge leap forward felt empowering, reminding me of a conversation I'd had recently with Rodrigo. When I'd told him I'd made the decision to have a baby on my own, using a sperm donor, he said, "You should change your name to Courage." Rodrigo had been raised in Mexico City and had moved to California seven years prior. He loved California's progressive vibe, and regularly marveled at my unconventional choices.

I laughed off his suggestion. "Who in the world would ever call themselves Courage?"

"Well, you should at least get a license plate that says: COURAGE," he insisted.

I blew him off at the time, but now, reflecting on my journey thus far, I understood his point. He was naming a quality in me that I rarely recognized or owned. But, having cleared the donor-choosing hurdle, now I could see it. When I wanted something, I did not sit around and twiddle my thumbs, I went after it. If that's what courageous people do, then yes, call me Courage.

More important, I was beginning to see my journey toward motherhood as something to be proud of. I wasn't a failure because I couldn't find a man to father a child with me. I was, instead, an empowered woman choosing to have a baby from a highly conscious place. I had thought out every aspect, worked through all my hang ups and fears, considered whether I was willing to make sacrifices in my lifestyle for my child. In another scenario, I may have gotten drunk and had reckless sex and gotten pregnant with a virtual stranger. I may have ended up in a loveless marriage just to have a baby, or simply given up on being a mother. I felt lucky that I lived during a time when women had a choice, when I could take clear, purposeful steps toward motherhood in my own way.

logistics of the first IUI

On top of picking a sperm donor, I'd also been masterminding the timing and logistics of the IUI. The way I figured it, I had only ten to fourteen days from the first day my period to get everything in order. I started off by scheduling a series of appointments. First stop: my gynecologist, to figure out my options for insemination.

"Well, you can call me the day you get a positive OPK, and I can try to fit you in. But if it lands on an evening or a weekend, I won't be able to help," she cautioned. "I'd make contact with a local midwife who does inseminations at home, in case the optimal time lands outside of my office hours."

Next stop: local midwife who did inseminations. It turned out that having a midwife come to my home would cost the same as seeing the doctor, and I loved the idea of hosting this rather intimate experience in the comfort and familiarity of my own bedroom. Plus the midwives would come to my house any time, day or night. I consulted with a midwife, Michelle, at her offices in Berkeley on day seven of my cycle. After we reviewed what I knew about my cycle and confirmed procedures for contacting her when it was go time, I left her office feeling reassured by her intricate knowledge of a woman's cycle and her concern for precise timing.

Then I scurried from Michelle's office across the bay to my third stop, Dr. Lee's in in San Francisco. She implemented a protocol that she believed would help bring fire to my pelvic region and belly, to ensure ovulation.

Since timing the IUI was the most critical part of the equation, I found another midwife, Kristin, who specialized in helping women gather and interpret data about their cycles, to pinpoint the optimal moment for insemination. Fourth stop: a Skype appointment, during which I told Kristin all about the herbs, the acupuncture, my diet, and my sessions with Chris. "I've also been tracking my BBT, my saliva ferning, and trying OPKs," I told her, "but my cycle is so irregular that I'm not getting anything consistent."

"Well, you are certainly doing a very thorough job, and doing much of what I would counsel you to do. There are few things we can add to help you figure out when to inseminate. They won't help you this cycle, but they will help you with the next few. Keep tracking your cycles and I can review your data and help you make sense of it for the next three months." Timing insemination is like trying to teach a computer to operate like a human's brain, except you're trying to understand and control the still quite mysterious intricacies of human conception. Kristin's assistance meant I wouldn't carry the burden alone; I'd have her years of experience along for the ride.

"Have you tried looking at your cervix with a speculum to see how it's changing over the month?" Kristin asked.

At one point in my life, this question would have knocked me over with its weirdness. But in Fertilityland, it was par for the course. I already knew that, nearing ovulation, the entrance to cervix, called the os, actually opens up. Supposedly you can see this with a speculum, and yes, I'd tried to look at mine. Despite some rather respectable yoga poses and gymnastic maneuvers, I saw nothing. Apparently, my cervix is camera shy. Maybe some women have a partner to help them track their cervical changes, but this was another thing I was going to have to figure out alone. Then again, imagine the awkward, lover-turned-gyno scenarios I'd be avoiding. Maybe alone was better after all?

As an alternative, Kristin suggested I feel my cervix daily to note its changes. "Right after your period, your cervix will feel as hard as your forehead. As you near ovulation, it will start to get softer, like the tip of your nose. And finally, when you are ovulating, it will be soft and squishy, like your chin." She did a little demo for me, placing her finger on each part of her face as she spoke and motioning for me to feel my own face. "You may also be able to feel that the opening is like a tiny pinhole when your cervix is hard. And when you are ovulating, there may be a clear opening that feels like a little dimple."

Kristin also suggested something called Lunaception. "Get some black-out curtains and make your room as dark as you possibly can. Keep it dark every single night, except when you should be ovulating. After a few months, your system may harmonize." Again, some might reject this suggestion out of hand as hippie-dippy mumbo jumbo, but I was willing to try anything. Besides, if she was right that I could trick my body into sync—how cool was that? "You are trying to emulate the moon's cycle and force your body to ovulate with the full moon."

When I mentioned my aggravating OPK results, Kristin didn't flinch. She responded like the woman she was—a calm, grounded midwife who had guided many women down this road. My story was no surprise to her. In her mind, the OPK tracked just one among many signs of ovulation. If I watched and tracked all signs, all at once, my body would give a complete picture. Given my OCD research tendencies, who could be better at ovulation tracking than me?

"If you really want an accurate fertility monitor," Kristin said, "you might want to invest in a monitor called the OvaCue, even though it's expensive. The great thing about is that it has both an oral and vaginal sensor for reading electrolyte levels that reflect hormone levels. It will accurately measure the changes in saliva leading up to ovulation and the vaginal sensor confirms ovulation." Then she added, "Don't forget about cervical fluid." As if I could forget? I'd been attempting to track for the last few months with no luck. Again, I didn't realize, or I refused to acknowledge, that my lack of cervical fluid was an indication that I was further along the road to menopause than I wanted to admit.

On Friday morning, day nine, I headed for stop five: a last-minute appointment with my OB/GYN for a peek at my ovaries. "You have maturing follicles on each ovary," she told me. "They are about fourteen to fifteen millimeters now. They need to grow to about twenty to twenty-four to ovulate. We assume they grow about one to two millimeters per day. Given that, you should ovulate by Monday or Tuesday."

I breathed a huge sigh of relief. *Good job, ovaries!* If I hadn't been on such a strict diet, I would have bought them a glass of Zinfandel to celebrate.

Later that afternoon, stop six brought me back to Chris, to make sure my body was operating in tiptop condition. Together we freed my pelvis of cold, damp qualities and ensured that my *Qi* was well organized and condensed, inviting for the Shen or light. The *Shen* is also referred to as the prenatal *Qi*, an essential ingredient to encourage new life to form inside me. I left Chris feeling energized and hopeful.

Having driven back and forth across the Bay multiple times in a few days, with insemination imminent, I was ready. Almost.

One cannot inseminate without sperm, of course. So while some folks prepare for conception with candles, a bottle of wine, and some favorite tunes set low on the Jambox, I set about my final task: order up a batch of sperm. I figured this would be the simplest of my tasks, since the bank was located in Palo Alto, about an hour from my house. Little did I know my samples were housed in Los Angeles. Suddenly the easy task of scheduling an in-office pick-up became a multi-level puzzle. The LA office would need to send my full order—five vials—to Palo Alto, then I could either pick up the vials I needed for this cycle at the Palo Alto office, or have them shipped to me. I wanted the sperm samples as early as Sunday, which would be day eleven of my cycle, however the office was closed on Sundays, and FedEx did not deliver on Saturday or Sunday. This meant I'd have to pick up the samples during business hours on Friday. But if insemination fell any time after Tuesday, my five-day storage tank would expire, as would my frozen specimens. The bank had access to seven-day storage tanks, but they used those only for shipments, not for in-office pick-ups. To complicate matters further, the representative on the phone—who I'm sure had walked clients thought this decision-making process countless times—offered no helpful suggestions, so I had to whip out my lawyer skills, figuring out the right questions, teasing out the information I needed to solve the problem. The most reasonable solution was to pick up the samples personally, in a seven-day tank, but the bank refused. They had a firm policy, about what I am not sure. About not allowing their clients to exercise the best solution? Eventually, after what felt like several infuriating hours on the phone, I decided to schedule the delivery via FedEx to arrive on Monday morning, crossing my fingers that ovulation wouldn't occur on Sunday. What other choice did I have?

With my sperm delivery set, I settled in for a nice long weekend of . . . tracking and waiting. More like obsessively tracking and anxiously waiting. While I silently begged my body not to ovulate before Monday, I honed in on every possible ovulation sign, frantic to know if it was honoring my request.

Remember that carnival game, the one where ducks slide by on a conveyor belt and people try to shoot them with fake rifles? Timing an IUI is a lot like that game, except the ducks travel in erratic, elliptical cycles while occasionally teleporting from place to place, and the bullets often die in midair. The variables in timing insemination had as much to do with pinpointing my body's optimal moment for delivery as they did with the lifespan of those all-important ingredients, the egg and sperm.

The IUI itself is a simple procedure in which a doctor or midwife inserts "washed sperm," or sperm extracted from semen, directly into the uterus to increase the chances of conception. While this delivery method eliminates some variables, like the sperm's long swim in search of and through the cervix, the goods being delivered—frozen sperm—spoil fast. When delivered the old-fashioned way, fresh sperm live three to five days inside a woman's body. Conversely, frozen, washed sperm, observed in a petri dish, live only twenty-four to forty-eight hours. Nobody knows how long frozen, washed sperm delivered via IUI, can live in a woman's body. Michelle and Kristin, both well-versed in home inseminations, believed that twenty-four to forty-eight hours was too generous an estimate. They told me to assume the sperm would only live for six to twenty-four hours.

And that's just half the timing equation. The lifespan of the egg is the other half. When a woman is young and fertile, her eggs are viable for twelve to twenty-four hours after ovulation. As women get older, the lifespan of an egg drastically diminishes, too, to about six to twelve hours after ovulation.

With the combined pressures of waiting, wondering, watching, and hoping bearing down on me, I spent the weekend trying to be calm and invite fertile thoughts. I diligently practiced Qigong and meditation every morning, and I avoided stressful or strenuous activities. In the pre-dawn hours of Sunday morning, I got up to use the bathroom. When I did, I noticed something different about my breasts. They felt full and tender, almost as if they'd gone up a bra size overnight. A former self would have been shaking her head at me right now. *Look at you, alone in your bathroom in the middle of the night, feeling yourself up.* But present-day me couldn't hear her. I was fully engulfed in ovulation-tracking mode. Immediately my gut said, *Your hormones just shifted radically.* I just wasn't sure if that meant I had already ovulated or if ovulation was imminent. With bleary eyes, I pulled out an OPK to see if I'd had the LH surge.

As I sat waiting the prescribed three minutes, I could barely keep my eyes open to read the very faint line that appeared, so faint that I assumed my LH levels had not yet spiked. *Maybe ovulation is coming,* my foggy mind hoped. Then again, it tossed in another possibility, *Maybe my LH spiked hours ago, and now I am catching it on the post-ovulation downslide.*

I climbed back in bed, tossing and turning the rest of the night, calculating and recalculating when I should be ovulating. The OPK was inconclusive, but my boobs felt so different. Perhaps if I had started testing with OPKs sooner in my cycle, I would have been able to compare the relative darkness of the test lines and determine whether my LH was surging or not. If I'd had a few months of data, I might have known whether this faint line was as good as it was going to get for me, or if there might be a darker line in my future.

When I'd met with Michelle, earlier that week, she'd told me to call her any time day or night if I thought I was ovulating, or if I was in any way unsure. But for some reason, I didn't call her. Maybe because the sperm hadn't arrived yet anyway?

Meanwhile, I treated my body like a chemical experiment, practicing the precise art of drinking just enough water, meaning enough so I could pee, but not so much that I would dilute the LH hormone detectable in my urine. In this way, I managed to pee on an OPK stick once every four hours, aching to see a darker line. No such luck. The lines continued to be so faint that I couldn't tell whether it was lighter or darker than the one before it. I whipped out a Sharpie and labeled each OPK with the date and time, then I lined them up on my bathroom vanity, in order, to compare lines. *I should probably call the midwife to discuss this,* I kept telling myself, followed by, *I should be able to figure this out on my own.*

Why didn't I call her? To this day, I cannot understand why I chose passivity, worried about bugging the midwife, instead of rallying to make the call.

On Monday morning, the sperm arrived early via FedEx. The samples came in a big box labeled "Human Specimen." What did the FedEx driver think he'd been transporting? Inside the box, I found a large metal tank filled with dry ice to keep the "human specimen" cryogenically frozen. I ceremoniously carried it upstairs, placing it in my meditation room, adorning it with pictures and relics of my teachers. Obviously, I'd take any good juju I could get.

I was hoping I would have time to do a mantra or some Qigong practice before the insemination, intending to create as much of a union between me and this sperm as possible. If it was true that a child picks its parents, I wanted to set out a strong beacon to attract a life in to me. Double-strong, actually, since I wasn't sure my frozen partner in this endeavor was capable of doing the same.

All day Monday, I continued the same routine, obsessively peeing on two or three brands of OPKs, checking my cervix, and taking my temperature. That afternoon, I went to Lowe's hardware to pick up some supplies for work I was having done on my house. While I was there, I started having a dull pain in my lower right pelvic region that I thought might be ovulation pain. Again I told myself that I should call the midwife. But I was relying on my OPKs, and they had still been so faint that I was hard pressed to say if they were getting darker or lighter. A nagging voice in my head kept telling me at least to call the midwife and check in, but I continued to sit on my hands. I felt so much pressure to get it right that my normal intuition and sensibility seemed to have gone out the window, taking my shot at conception with it.

The next morning's OPK stick showed no line at all. Dread washed over me. *Oh, god, why did I wait to call the midwife?*

In hindsight, I knew the moment had passed. I was likely my most fertile late Saturday night, when I felt my breasts change. Nevertheless, I rushed to my computer to email the midwife before heading out to teach my weekly Qigong class. Despite my mental state before class, I pulled it together, as I always did, to show up for my students. No matter what stirred up in my personal life, teaching called me to drop the crap, become present, and return to clarity. But soon after class, life, that eternal jokester, pressed the chaos button again. As I arrived home, intending to call Michelle, I was met by my construction guys who were starting a new project in my bedroom. After answering their million questions and showing them the supplies I had bought at Lowe's, finally, around noon I called Michelle, giving her the download of information.

"Sounds like you probably missed it," she said. My heart sank. Again, the frustration. *How could I have missed it? Why didn't I try calling sooner?* "But for the sake of not wasting a cycle, let's still try one vial," she said. "But we've got to do it ASAP. I'm unavailable till later this afternoon. Do you mind if my business associate, Rebecca, comes? She can be there in forty-five minutes."

Just as I was telling Michelle to send Rebecca, my carpenter interrupted, "Hey, Sarah. I'm gonna go for lunch. I'll be back in about thirty minutes, and then I'll start working on the closet in your bedroom."

My *room?* After weeks waiting for their schedule to free up, why did they need my room *today?* I briefly considered sending the construction crew home, but I didn't want to miss my chance to get this project started. I'd done enough missing chances for one day. Instead, I called my roommate to ask if I could use her room. "Of course," she said. "Make yourself comfortable and don't even worry for one second."

As I prepped the room for the midwife's arrival, carrying the sperm tank in and placing pictures of my spiritual teachers, calling on their wisdom and enlightenment to grace this experience, the irony hit me. I had wanted to normalize the experience of artificial insemination as much as possible by giving it some modicum of familiarity and intimacy, but now it would happen in my roommate's bed, with a midwife I'd never met, accompanied by the soundtrack of a construction crew doing demo work in my bedroom closet. Was this the first clue that I would control next to nothing about my journey toward motherhood? I grabbed a blanket and pillows from my room, to make my roommate's space feel more like my own and, honestly, to avoid any seepage or spills on her bed.

Despite the weirdness, the insemination ended up being a lovely experience.

Rebecca was about my age, with a calm soothing demeanor. I led her up to my roommate's room, and she spoke softly and slowly as she asked me to recap everything that had happened. Because I'd been going non-stop all morning, I was ready to move at lightning speed, speaking in a rushed hurried fashion, but Rebecca's pace was infectious and I managed to slow down. We went through the fertility signs again. "On Friday my OB/GYN spotted two maturing follicles—one on each ovary." I told her about the feeling in my breasts on Saturday night, and the ovulation pain on Monday, as well as the faint OPK line that had completely disappeared.

Rebecca counterbalanced my urgency with her soothing demeanor and soft voice, "Well, it sounds like you ovulated at least once, but maybe you still need to ovulate on the other side."

I almost gasped out loud when she said this. *Maybe this is perfect timing for the second ovulation?*

As Rebecca opened the tank, I heard a whisper of pressure released and a trickle of cold steam rose out of the opening. She pulled a long metal pole up out of the tank and removed a tiny vial of sperm attached to the bottom. The vial was smaller than my pinky finger. *This teeny vial encasing an even teenier sperm ice cube cost eight hundred bucks?* How many men spilled gallons of that stuff over a lifetime, with no regard to its value? And yet, one infinitesimal drop might get me pregnant. It seemed well worth the cost.

Rebecca placed the frosty vial inside a hand towel and held the towel in her hand. About a minute later, she unwrapped the vial and handed it to me. "Rub it between your palms for about five minutes," she instructed. I hadn't really thought about how we would defrost the vial, but this low-tech method surprised me.

As I held the vial between my hands, I spoke a silent prayer. *Please, let me have a baby. Please, please, please. I promise that I will love it so carefully and consciously. I will shower it with love and be the best mom I can be. Please, please, please!*

While I held the vial, Rebecca reviewed the paperwork accompanying the sperm sample. She remarked at the amazing motility and count for the sperm. "As good as it gets," she said. "Would you like to look at the sperm under the microscope to make sure it's alive and kicking?"

"How would we do that?" I asked.

"I'd have to take out a tiny drop to put on a slide for you to look at." I looked again at the miniature vial, at best about quarter full. I couldn't imagine losing one precious drop. "No, that's okay," I said.

"Okay, then let's get you set up. Lie down on the bed for me. I'm going to place some pillows under your hips and then I'll prepare the specimen."

I complied, then Rebecca took the vial from me and drew the specimen up into a syringe, diligently sucking up every errant droplet at the bottom of the vial and in the cap. Then she placed the speculum and slowly inserted a small tube catheter up through my cervix and released the sperm into my uterus. I shed a few tears right at the moment the catheter passed into my uterus, but otherwise felt calm. Were they tears of joy, fear, sadness, loneliness, or a mix of all of them? I had thought I might suddenly question what I was doing or feel a huge surge of loneliness about this very clinical means of conception, but that never happened. I simply knew I was doing what I had to do.

Rebecca waited a moment, explaining, "If I withdraw the catheter too quickly, the sample could spill back out." Then she pulled the catheter out and packed up to go, instructing me to remain lying down for at least thirty minutes. "Let's hope we got lucky for a second ovulation," she said as she closed the bedroom door behind her.

I breathed in and relaxed into the bed. I had expected the whole thing to feel like a momentous occasion, but instead it felt anti-climactic, quite mundane and straightforward. I laid in my roommate's bed for nearly an hour, diligently singing the mantra for White Tara, Divine Mother and Wish Grantor, and prayed for a healthy, happy baby, while the construction crew's pounding and sawing echoed down the hall from my bedroom. I tried to forgive myself for not calling the midwife sooner and hoped for the best.

A few hours later, pain gripped the left side of my pelvis, starting out dull and reaching a crescendo with a sharp stab at around 5:00 P.M. *Second ovulation?* I wondered. *Maybe someone was looking out for me after all? Maybe I'd actually timed insemination just right, to avoid twins?* As the dreaded two-week wait—the recommended timespan between insemination and the first pregnancy test—began, I vacillated between feeling like the biggest idiot for not calling the midwife and feeling brilliant for instinctively avoiding becoming a single mom with twins. One moment I was certain I was pregnant, and the next I was convinced I had no chance. I would later learn this incessant, dichotomous thinking wasn't unique to me. The Internet is home to numerous chat rooms, blogs, and websites dedicated to surviving the anxiety-provoking two-week wait.

babies are dukkha

wo weeks later, my alarm sounded its pleasant chime, waking me out of a fitful sleep at 5:00 A.M. I was up unusually early to catch a plane to a meditation retreat in Olympia, just outside Seattle, led by Luang Por Jamnian, a Thai forest monk. I shuffled into the bathroom to pee, blurry eyed and groggy, but I snapped to attention when I looked and saw it: blood. I wasn't pregnant. My heart sank a little, but I wasn't crushed. The start of my period simply confirmed that I had in fact timed the insemination incorrectly, but it didn't mean I was incapable of conceiving. I shook it off and grabbed my luggage, pulling out the pregnancy tests and the mountain of supplements that I would have used if I had gotten a positive pregnancy test, and leaving in all my paraphernalia for tracking my cycle instead.

I dreaded the logistics of taking my temperature and using oral and vaginal sensors in a big dorm room, with a bunch of strangers. Worse still, when given the option of staying in a regular cabin, snoring cabin, or "noble silence" cabin, my friends had opted for noble silence, presuming the nomenclature meant people in that cabin not only wouldn't talk but wouldn't snore. I had disagreed about that last bit, but I signed on anyway. So now I'd be stuck in a noble silence cabin where my very un-noble beeping monitors would be highlighted by the lack of conversation and noise. But I was determined to do it anyway. I didn't want to interrupt Project Baby, nor did I want to miss this opportunity to practice with Luang Por Jamnian for seven days.

Through my Qigong practice, I'd become open to and curious about all religious traditions, and I'd always been drawn to Buddhism as a way to learn more about the workings of my mind. Back in 2005, when I'd been going through a particularly hard period, Chris had suggested I find a Theravada monk with whom to study *vipassana*, the awareness practice out of which the now-popular practice of mindfulness evolved. To my delight, I discovered that Luang Por Jamnian was coming from Thailand to the Bay Area to lead a twelve-day retreat. By the end of those twelve days, I'd gained a clear view into the unclean motivations behind even my most seemingly innocuous actions.

For example, the retreat had been filled with a gaggle of eager students, all of whom were anxiously waiting their turn to ask a question. So when I had a question, I'd need to wait hours, sometimes days, to ask. But that time allowed me to pause. Rather than just blurting out my question the moment it came to mind, I had to sit, pondering why I wanted to ask my question. That alone was revelatory. Hidden inside every question I found something else—a subtle desire to show how much I knew about the topic, or a cry for attention. Once I saw this tendency, I sat mute for the remainder of the retreat, forever changed in my ability to ask questions. This humbling realization gave me a firsthand experience of the ego and *self* as distinct from my true nature. By the end of the retreat, I also felt like the proverbial duck, with water washing off my back unable to stick. I could not muster an ounce of anxiety and instead watched as even the most disturbing topics of conversation passed by not causing the slightest distress.

When I returned from my first retreat with Luang Por Jamnian, Chris was so intrigued by my transformation that the following year, when Jamnian returned to the US, Chris attended the retreat with me. As the years went on, more and more of my fellow Qigong students had started attending his retreats as well. For health reasons, Jamnian had not been able to travel to the US for several years, so now Chris, two of his other serious students, and I were eager to see him again.

Although Luang Por Jamnian often taught long, complicated lessons about Buddhist scriptures, the kernel of his teaching was simple: practice the Middle Way. In short, this means learning to notice the mind drifting toward liking or disliking, and committing to return the mind to the neutral state, which is devoid of any preferences or aversions. When I'd practiced this on past retreats, it had led me to profound clarity, a state in which I felt complete equanimity. In this state I was unaffected by the pushes and pulls of normal life. Indeed the "knowing" to which Chris had referred when he was helping me decide whether or not to have a baby was a key component of the Middle Way.

As is often the case in spiritual and religious traditions, Theravada Buddhism is surrounded by its own amount of legend and what some might call superstition. Luang Por Jamnian, considered to be fully enlightened, or a living Buddha, was a revered monk of legendary status in the Theravada tradition. For one, as a small boy, around the age of six, he began spontaneously reciting Buddhist scriptures—a skill said to arise when someone has reincarnated from a previous master. As a result, people believed that Luang Por Jamnian could grant wishes, heal disease, manifest prosperity, and help people in various other ways. In Thailand and Asia, people pilgrimage thousands of miles to receive his blessings. He often receives thousands of people a day.

Even my lawyer mind had to affirm Luang Por Jamnian's abilities, as I'd had my own experience of his healing power. When I had gone to see him the first time, I was still living with nearly constant pain. Sitting for hours at a time, for multiple days in a row was causing horrible headaches. During my private interview with him, I asked him to tell me more about his role as a healer. It was this fascination with healers that had compelled me to study medical anthropology in college. "No, sorry. I don't do that anymore," he explained through the translator. But after I left my private interview, I returned to my room and shook violently in my bed for over thirty minutes. When the tremors finally ceased, my physical pain and headache were gone. As the retreat continued, my pain would start to return from time to time. But then I would notice Jamnian smiling and nodding at me in a knowing way, and my pain would disappear instantly. How could I question the veracity of his legendary healing after that?

This time around, I was eager to ask Luang Por Jamnian's for help getting pregnant. Maybe he could see something in my karmic past that needed to be forgiven or realized? Or he'd simply remove some impediment or blockage that needed to be released? I wasn't sure what he could do, really. I'd welcome any help I could get. But before I could receive this powerful healing, I'd have to endure an extremely rustic, water logged retreat center, which seemed hell bent on pulling me out of the Middle Way, into aversion and disliking.

First, the dining experience dug at me. Originally the teachings were scheduled to take place in a converted barn, but the freezing cold and damp conditions forced us to consolidate all activities into the dining hall. Logistically, this meant the dining hall was split in two—half of it storing our rugs and pillows for teachings, the other half used as our eating space, with long, plastic tables squished so tightly together only a waif could pass comfortably. Hot water stood on one side of the room, food in another corner, utensils and plates in the other. Once you made your rounds and sat down, if you forgot something, you had to suck in your belly and squeeze between rows of chairs and tables. Ever the strategists, my friend Genevieve and I decided to manage meal time and our frustrations by teaming up, cutting in half the number of trips we'd have to make through the tables. To make matters worse, every meal, and I mean *every* meal, was Thai food, catered by a local restaurant, with the menu limited to dishes they could serve easily en masse. I love Thai food, but this was more like "cafeteria Thai," and let's be honest, there's only so much Pad Thai a person can eat in a week.

Second, the notorious Pacific Northwest rain eroded my mood, beginning on the second day and continuing thereon. My boots leaked, forcing me to create an intricate system of wearing already wet socks while walking to and from my cabin, then switching to dry socks once I arrived inside. I yearned for respite, but thanks to the constant downpours outside, my only options were to perch in my horrible, coffin-like bed in silence, or to hang out in the overly crowded and always chaotic dining hall.

Many of the other seventy-odd participants seemed to take this all in stride, on their best behavior, grateful to be in the presence of this great teacher. But I, for one, was grouchy and irritable, not light and mindful, which darkened my mood all the more.

From the outset, I was preoccupied with my plan to ask Jamnian about my desire to get pregnant. I listened to each of his talks through this lens. Many times he repeated, "This lifetime brings only suffering." He told stories of families that had come to him distraught by the fact that their children didn't obey them, or complaining about their children's difficult lives. He was happy to be a monk, unable to bear children of his own. It was clear that to Luang Por Jamnian having a child only brought suffering. As I sat pondering his talks, I agreed that if people really thought it through logically they would not decide to have children. Despite all the very good reasons not to have a baby, my heart yearned for one. I was willing to accept a certain degree of suffering to reap the joys.

Maybe I should have heard Luang Por Jamnian's position on babies and changed my questions for him. But I didn't. I forged ahead, convinced that he would be able to see what, if anything, was in my way karmically, or that he would pull out his revered healing skills to cure me. A friend, childless after three years of trying, had also planned to ask him about what might be blocking her from having a child, but she backed out after getting the gist of Jamnian's thoughts on the topic: Babies are *dukkha*, the Pali word for suffering. Undeterred—or perhaps headstrong and unwaveringly focused on my project—I planned to ask for help anyway.

Looking back, I see how much power I gave to Luang Por Jamnian and my hopes for this meeting. As I sat in a small, dark, narrow hallway, waiting to enter the small interview room, I was surrounded by two students who were debating the nuances of the stages of enlightenment. One student, who I found particularly annoying, was convinced that Luang Por Jamnian had gotten a detail about the final stages of enlightenment wrong. "He has to be wrong," she said pointing out what might have seemed like an inconsistency. "I'm going to confront him. Someone needs to nail him down and get him to give us the right answer." The irony was too much for me—this debating of the final stage of enlightenment, when she was exuding enough dislike and anger to fill the entire hallway and beyond. What's more, Luang Por Jamnian had repeatedly explained that it was impossible to contemplate or comprehend the stages of enlightenment with a normal mind. They are so beyond our ken that only one who has reached enlightenment can contemplate the nuance of the final stages.

My irritation grew as their debate heated up. *Notice dislike. This is anger arising*, I told myself, feebly attempting to apply the teachings. But the neutrality of the Middle Way was far beyond my grasp at the moment. I was too preoccupied with my upcoming conversation to gain control of my mind when I needed to most. But at least I was aware of my dislike and knew that I was far from enlightenment. My hallmate was ready to wage war against Luang Por Jamnian, because she thought she knew the stages of enlightenment better than him.

Eventually, the enlightenment avenger changed topics, complaining, "And he is always running so late. Someone needs to enforce the time limit. He needs boundaries, and I'm not afraid to enforce them." Now she was killing me. Her blatant disrespect of an enlightened master floored me. But, more to the point, I was also about to ask a very important question, seek help on a matter so dear to my heart. Why was she here now, determined to restore order and justice by being the timekeeper? Couldn't she trust that an enlightened master could decide how much time was appropriate for each person? People waited a lifetime to speak to him. But more importantly, if he and I were in the middle of something, I didn't want my time being cut short because *she'd* decided it was time to move on.

When I could stand no more, I silently willed the woman to go away. But that didn't work, so I mustered up as much "mindfulness of speech" as I could to ask her, ever so gently, to bring her debate down the hall. Still she lurked, insisting to the designated time keeper, "Someone needs to enforce boundaries with that man."

When I was finally escorted into the tiny room to see Luang Por Jamnian, at least twenty minutes late, I was flustered. Luang Por Jamnian sat in a chair far too small for him, engulfed in layers of saffron robes, weighted down by over forty kilos of weights, amulets, and trinkets in order to remind him that there is suffering that needs constantly to be released. He beamed a huge smile when I walked in, either recognizing me from previous retreats, or more likely shining his constant beacon of joy. Luang Por Jamnian was always transmitting a blissful state, and if you paid attention you could jump on the wave of joy. Unfortunately, today was a different story.

To Luang Por Jamnian's left, a young monk sat on a mattress on the floor. He sat beside Jamnian wherever he went, for seven days, never uttering a word, simply abiding quietly in equanimity. I yearned for an ounce of his peacefulness. To Luang Por Jamnian's right sat a Thai man, Pat, who was acting as a translator. Pat was a lovely man, but the English speakers at these retreats never knew whether Pat's translation was accurate, because Thai speakers were often correcting his translations for him and growing increasingly agitated as they listened to his translation. It was hard to tell whether the gap in translation was because Pat's English was limited or because he was adding his own impressions and embellishments. Regardless, I was sure something was getting lost in translation. Usually I didn't care. Jamnian's energy didn't need a literal translation. But today was different.

I sat down on the cold, hard chair across from Jamnian and opened my mouth to speak, but I immediately burst into tears. I managed to blurt out some string of words between my tears. "I really want a baby, but I am having problems getting pregnant. My Western doctors have said that it might be impossible. But I don't believe them. I'm not willing to give up yet." Pat looked a bit shocked and worried as I spoke, but I forged ahead, wanting to get out all my thoughts before relinquishing my message to Pat. "Can you see what is getting in my way karmically, or what might be preventing me from having a baby? Can you see anything that is blocking me? Can you help me get pregnant?"

Pat turned back to face Luang Por Jamnian. Pat relayed what I had said to Luang Por Jamnian, then I waited while Luang Por Jamnian responded to Pat, who muttered little sounds of comprehension and surprise, while I tried to gain some control over my sobs. I planted my feet on the ground, using breath to sink into my body, but I was so tense it had little effect. Finally, Pat turned back to me and clasped his hands in his lap, a relieved look on his face as if he had feared Luang Por Jamnian might be stumped by my question, and he was pleased that Jamnian had come back with such a satisfactory answer. "Umm, yes, he said, 'Don't worry if you can't have babies, they are only *dukkha* anyways.'"

What? He must have gotten the translation wrong, I told myself. *I need to clarify my question.* While trying to fight back a full-blown sobbing attack, I stammered, "No, no. I don't know if it is actually impossible for me to get pregnant. Western doctors say it might be, but I don't believe them. I still want to try." I reiterated again for good measure, "It is difficult, but not necessarily impossible. I want his help. Can you see anything that is blocking me?"

Again, I waited patiently while my message was translated back and forth. Pat turned to me again with elation, "Ah, yes. He said again that 'babies are just *dukkha*. So, don't worry. You've escaped the misery!'" Despite the horror on my face, he continued, "He says that so many people come to him about problems with their children. 'My child is disobeying me. My child doesn't want to do what I tell him to do.' Jamnian sees that babies are really just suffering, and it's not something he can get involved in."

Impossible, I thought. *There is no way an enlightened master is saying this. The problem must be in the translation*, I insisted. Jamnian seemed to talk for ages to Pat, but Pat's responses to me were short and curt. Something wasn't lining up. I gave it one final shot, trying again to clarify, but I got the same response: Congratulations, babies are *dukkha*. Their patience in the matter only made it worse. Despair crept through my whole body.

Luang Por Jamnian tried to impart another teaching on me, maybe simply in an attempt to move the conversation forward, since I was growing more and more agitated. But I had shut down. I was so angry at Jamnian for refusing to help me. I made no attempts to hide my displeasure, folding my arms across my chest with a big huff. I may have even interrupted him or tried to contradict him. Rage scrambled my brain so badly I was struggling to comprehend what Jamnian was saying. And then it happened: a knock on the door. "Your time's up," the enlightenment debater's voice said, keeping good on her promise to hold Jamnian to a tight schedule. But at this point, I was too exasperated to care. I flew out of the room, blowing past the shocked faces of students in the hallway, tears streaming down my face. Most people leave these interviews elated and buoyant, blasted by his brightness. I can only imagine what those people in the hallway thought of me.

I ran out into the rain, headed toward a lake at the other end of the retreat center, letting the caged up sobs unleash. No, I decided, nothing had been lost in translation. He could see that I would never have a baby, so he was trying to help me get over it. Why had I ever asked him for help? I should have known his opinion about babies and *dukkha*. An hour later, Chris came and found me. Immediately, he could see that the interview hadn't gone well.

"I knew your interview could be either the panacea or cause for complete devastation. What's going on? Where are you at?" he asked.

I explained what had happened, and Jamnian's adamant opinion that babies are suffering. I was gasping for breath between sobs as I spoke. "I'm not totally sure that my question was translated properly, but now I'm terrified that he can see that I'm not supposed to get pregnant, so he's trying to prepare me."

"You don't know that," Chris reassured me. "I would assume more that it's an area in which he doesn't feel comfortable helping. I get it. Having a baby takes you further away from practice. For him, the only path is toward enlightenment. Life needs to be simple to attain enlightenment. That's why monks live in a monastery where they don't have to worry about food, shelter, and clothing.

They take vows to simplify life so completely that they actually have a shot at enlightenment. He doesn't understand why anyone would want a family. He's been in a monastery since he was a young boy. The idea of getting married or having kids is completely foreign to him."

"Are you sure?" I questioned. "I thought that once someone reached his level of enlightenment he could basically see into my mind, my karma, my future?"

"He can see into your deep consciousness. When you told me you wanted to ask him for help, I hoped that he would look into your mind and point out any obstacles in your path. He may have looked and seen that there was nothing much blocking you. Who knows? But instead, he gave you a very Buddhist answer—that all life is suffering. And on some level, he's right. But that shouldn't stop you from having a child if you want one."

I spent the rest of the break trying to calm myself down and take in Chris's words. When we returned to the meditation hall a few hours later, Jamnian began to tell a story. "There were two earthworms. One lived in the Deva realm, a heaven-like realm, and no longer needed to eat, sleep, or worry about any basic needs. He craved nothing, and he had no worries or cares in the world. The other worm lived in an outhouse, amongst the defecation and filth. He was happy, however, because he did not have to look for food. He could just constantly eat the poop that was in never-ending supply. He could indulge himself as much as he wanted.

"One day, the Deva Worm went to visit the Outhouse Worm. The Outhouse Worm asked the Deva Worm about his life. The Deva Worm explained, 'Life is amazing. There is no outhouse, no mess. I don't need food, but if I want it I can have it on demand. I no longer need to sleep. There is just endless happiness unlike anything I could have ever imagined.'

"The Outhouse Worm was puzzled. 'But, life in the outhouse is amazing. I don't have to think about what to eat. There is constantly food—it's an endless supply without any hassles. I don't have to think about it in order for it to appear. And, I enjoy sleeping, why would I want to stay awake all the time?' The Deva

Worm kept trying to explain how great it was to be in the heavenly realm, but the Outhouse Worm could not comprehend it. He was attached to his outhouse world."

About halfway through the story, I suspected it was for me. Luang Por Jamnian explained, "People often come to me with requests. These requests make no sense while I am sitting in the boundless happiness of nirvana. The Deva Worm can't make sense of the Outhouse Worm's life. And vice versa. The Outhouse Worm cannot understand how and why the Deva Worm wants for nothing. When people ask for things that from my perspective cause suffering, I can't get involved." And then, just in case I was confused about whether the story truly was for me, he added, "Being born into this world causes suffering, so I stay out of anything to do with babies."

Immediately, I felt my heart burst open. I had mistaken his response as a lack of care. But in this moment, I could feel his intense love and concern. I could also feel the sting of my behavior—I'd been disrespectful during our meeting, lost in my suffering. I needed to ask for forgiveness.

I spent the next twenty-four hours stewing in remorse, plotting my request for forgiveness. I could approach him and ask for a forgiveness ceremony, or I could try to send a note, but that would have to be translated by someone. Neither of those options seemed logistically plausible or appealing. The next day, a woman approached Luang Por Jamnian as he sat at his table eating lunch. She knelt before him and asked for a blessing. Jamnian began chanting as a small group gathered like puppies around a food bowl, hoping to get in on the goods. Jamnian had said many times that he knows what is in our hearts without us having to say anything, so I tried an experiment. I sat close by during the blessing, clearly and loudly saying in my head, *I'm sorry. I appreciate and respect your response to me.* Over and over, I repeated this in my head, filled with sorrow, respect, and love.

At the end of the blessing, Luang Por Jamnian walked over to me and bonked me on the head with a staff type thing he carried around. As far as I knew, it contained amulets and sacred items for blessings. With a giant grin on his face, he looked me straight in the eye and said, in English, "I love you. You love me. I love you. You love me. Happy, happy." A wave of relief washed over me. Some may be more cynical than I, but I was confident he had heard my penance and forgiven me.

As the retreat ended, Luang Por Jamnian's message resonated: choosing a child means choosing not to pursue enlightenment as it is viewed by the Theravada sect of Buddhism. I didn't doubt that parenthood would provide unlimited opportunities for self-reflection and self-improvement. But having a child would complicate my life, which would mean stepping off a certain spiritual path my other friends would continue walking without me. Motherhood did not mean giving up spiritual practice in general though. What better way to challenge myself continually to return to the Middle Way than changing diapers and cleaning up puke? I could think of no better gift to my child than striving to reside in the Middle Way through the ups and downs of motherhood.

I was at a fork in the road, and Jamnian had been trying his hardest to signal the significance of my choices. Perhaps he was testing my resolve: *If you're going to do this thing that creates so much suffering, you better be damn certain that you know what you are doing and still want it.* I still wanted it. This was not a passing whim; it was my truth. As much as I admired Luang Por Jamnian and my other teachers, I had to stay true to my own life's path, unshaken by the opinions of others, even my revered masters. I smiled and thanked Luang Por Jamnian for giving me the opportunity to reaffirm my commitment. Yes, babies are *dukkha*, but I was ready for the sacrifice. I was more certain than ever that I wanted to be a mother.

more disappointment

I got home from the retreat with Luang Por Jamnian at 8:00 P.M. on Sunday, and demolition of my kitchen began the following morning, at 8:00 A.M. Though a good friend and kitchen cabinet designer was making my cabinets, I was acting as my own general contractor to save money, managing the workers, ordering all the products, scheduling the various construction crews, and organizing the order in which everything needed to be installed. I knew I had a pattern of taking on too much, but it was too late to hire a contractor, so I put on my virtual hardhat and got to work.

Between phone calls and construction-related errands, I continued the crazy-making task of tracking my body's fertility signs. As I suspected, the noble silence cabin had not made data gathering easy. The loud beeping noises on my BBT thermometer and OvaCue monitor were too embarrassing so I barely used them. So when I scheduled my second IUI, calling the sperm bank to place an order and putting the midwife on notice, I was mostly guessing.

As if to make up for lost time, upon my return home, instead of doing an OPK test once a day, precisely twenty-four hours apart, I began peeing on OPK sticks—three different brands—every single time I used the bathroom. I was *not* going to miss my window of opportunity this time.

Again the OPK sticks produced faint lines, next to impossible to distinguish. At least this time, I knew better than to wait for the lines to darken. I also knew better than to wait to call Michelle. On Wednesday morning, June 13, I thought my cervix felt soft and open, so I called her before dawn. I thought it might be premature, but I didn't want to miss the ovulation window. When she arrived around 8:00 A.M., she suggested that we check whether my cervix was ready by trying to insert the catheter before thawing and opening the sperm vial. I agreed.

"I can't get the catheter past the os of your cervix," she explained. "Your cervix is not open enough." Had we missed ovulation and my cervix was closing now, or were we too early? "Do you know how long your cervix stays open before and after ovulation?" she asked.

"I have no idea," I confessed. "I still haven't gotten a handle on what my cervix is doing." The voices in my head immediately started chattering about how I wasn't doing a good enough job.

After much deliberation, Michelle and I decided she would come back in twelve hours to check the progress of my cervix. It was guesswork based on too little information, but she seemed confident.

For those next twelve hours, I obsessively continued to check my cervix and pee on OPK sticks. Each time, I would label them with the date and time, then lay them out in a neat row with their predecessors, for comparison. Then I would gather them up and hide them in the top drawer of my vanity, to spare my roommate and the construction workers. After several rounds of cervix checks, it seemed like it my cervix might have been getting softer, but the OPKs were still confusing. When Michelle returned that night, the catheter passed with no problem. Michelle exclaimed happily, "That means we have a good chance of catching ovulation." Although people think you can inseminate after ovulation, in fact you can't. The sperm must be inside the uterus at the time of ovulation, ready to meet the egg. As Michelle thawed the vial of sperm and completed the IUI, I crossed my fingers that we had inseminated in time.

Though the timing seemed perfect, I still opted to do a second IUI in eighteen hours. When Michelle returned, however, my cervix was closed again. "I hope that means we timed the first one perfectly," I said. "Hopefully I just saved myself $800 by using only one vial of sperm." The sperm bank would allow me to return an unopened vial to storage for use when I needed it next.

I awoke the next morning, and reached for my thermometer. If I had ovulated, my resting temperature should have risen, due to the presence of progesterone. No luck, though. My temp remained the same. My brain immediately began spitting out data, buoying my hopes. *I hadn't been able to take my BBT on retreat, so maybe this seemingly low temperature was due to poor data.* Then I used the OvaCue vaginal monitor, looking for ovulation confirmation, but it too failed to yield a positive result. Either I hadn't ovulated or I simply wasn't producing progesterone.

Discouraged but unwilling to give in, I rode up and down hope's yo-yo string for two weeks, waiting to take a pregnancy test. Alas, the test was a big fat negative, and my period followed shortly afterward. I called Chris in tears and asked for a session.

Over the past few months, my sessions with Chris had been focused mainly on making my reproductive system as healthy as possible—removing cold and swelling from my pelvic region. However, a few weeks prior, Chris had hinted that I had some emotional issues that might be impeding my bodily systems and preventing me from conceiving. I was hoping that he might be able to work on these blocks during this session.

Chris met me at my house, and I led him to my spare room, which I used as a treatment room. The session started like any other, with me lying on my back, fully supported by pillows and other props. With my body fully supported, I felt myself starting to let go of tensions and habitual contractions all over my body: my jaw, around my eyes, and my gut. With this, my mind calmed, and I was lulled into a dreamlike state. Chris placed his hand ever so softly over my solar plexus, "Can you sense the emotion in this area?" he asked. Before I could answer, I started breathing heavily, my throat fluttered, and I started to cry. "What are you feeling now?" he asked.

I paused for a moment to tune into the sensations in that area. "I think I am feeling anger, but I'm not sure."

"Okay, stay with those sensations and emotions." Slowly, the sensations started to intensify. My breathing became jagged and I felt strange pushes and pulls as my body flashed between waves of heat and intense chills. My jaw clenched, and I gnawed my teeth together. Soon, a series of images started flitting through my mind, horrible images of hurting my mother. The kinds of images you would never want to admit to anyone. I was overcome by intense anger and hatred as my breath became more and more erratic.

"What's going on now?" Chris asked. At first, I was hesitant to admit what I was feeling, worried what this experience said about me. But I also implicitly trusted Chris, so I began to explain, "I am experiencing intense hatred of my mother. The images are incredibly graphic and violent. They won't go away." I hesitated before I continued, not sure I was willing to admit what was happening, even to Chris. "I keep trying to kill my mother. I am seeing myself ripping my mother apart, limb-by-limb. It feels horrible and depraved."

My mom and I had never had an easy relationship, but I knew I loved her. Ever since I was a young girl, we were often at odds with each other. I had no tolerance for her frequent yelling and anger. As an adult, she had disagreed with many of my decisions, leaving me feeling unsupported. But my feelings now made no sense to me. They were foreign, out of proportion to any anger I had ever felt toward her.

"Okay, stay with that," Chris said reassuringly. He wasn't fazed by my emotions, which allowed me to stay present to what was happening. "And what does the physical contraction in that area feel like?"

I struggled to find the words to map my visceral sensations. I could feel an empty hole and a strange area of contraction to the right side of my solar plexus. I struggled with the words as the sensations got stronger. I felt so overcome with raw emotion that my chest heaved up and down exaggeratedly. I couldn't speak or narrate what was happening, in part because there were no words for it, but also because the experience was too overwhelming to allow me to multitask. I worked hard at staying completely present to the experience. A series of hot, cold, and burning waves coursed through my body, alternating with the sensation that my organs were being ripped in different directions. Just when I thought I could no longer take the intensity of the physical sensations and images, the violent fantasies came to an end. In their place, I began to see lovely, soft images of my mother being kind and loving. My breath began to smooth out and a softness washed over me.

Chris must have been able to sense what was happening because just then he asked me to think about my mother as a child. I thought about her background, growing up during World War II in England and the Depression that followed. I could picture her then, a sweet girl being shuttled around from house to house to avoid air raids, or running into the bomb shelter in the backyard. I could feel her fear and anxiety. I called to mind her mother's death, from breast cancer, shortly before I was born. How hard it must have been, coddling an infant while mourning the loss of her own mother. I was taken aback by the selflessness of her love and the sacrifices she'd made raising me.

As my empathy and tenderness toward her increased, the parts of my body that had previously felt like they were ripping apart now felt harmonious and light. I luxuriated in the love and warmth I felt toward my mother. The gaping hole in my solar plexus now felt full. Something had changed radically in my over-all sensation of my body.

After a few minutes, as the fullness too started to subside, I reached equilibrium. I cautiously asked Chris, "What was *that?* What just happened?" I had no idea I was capable of such horrible thoughts and images of my mother. I knew we didn't get along some of the time, but *that* was crazy.

"What do you feel about your mother now?" he probed.

"I feel love and kindness toward her," I said. "It must be so difficult to be a mother." I paused as I marveled at what it takes to be a mother. "I think I'm only just comprehending what a truly selfless act motherhood is. And I see how much my mother must care for me, even though it's sometimes difficult for her to express."

"Good," he replied. "It's important to realize that those were not feelings about your actual mother. It's easy for you to associate them with your mother, even though what you're feeling has nothing to do with her. You've personified those feelings into images of your mother, but they are actually feelings you have toward yourself as a mother. You've been carrying a certain charge of anger in your system. It lives in your tissues, unassociated with any subject or object, even though you've tied it to many things, including your mother and your idea of yourself as a mother. I wanted you to go through this process and see these feelings so that you could discharge them, transform them, and move past them. They were putting a certain drag on your system. Normally, I wouldn't lead you directly into them, I'd let you slowly work on each piece, but you want a baby and they were getting in your way."

I knew well what Chris was talking about. One of the most incredible aspects of Qigong for me had been the ability to have intense emotional experiences that were unassociated with a particular trigger. Many times in class I would suddenly be overcome by sadness or anger. Chris would counsel, "Stay with the raw sensations. Don't create a story around it or grasp to give it meaning. Let it just be emotions moving through." He would later explain how the tissues, muscle patterns, and lymph in the body could hold on to emotions. "When you do energetic practice, you can move fluids and change old muscular patterns that can cause stuck emotions to come rushing to the surface. It can feel like getting hit with a Mack truck of emotions. But if you let them pass through, then you have a chance to transform or create lasting change. If you try, however, to give what's happening meaning or associate certain events with the experience, you create a grasping and will likely recreate the emotions."

In this case, Chris had helped me experience the emotions, and it had certainly felt like a discharge. "How is this related to my ability to get pregnant?" I asked, still trying to make sense of what had just happened.

"The anger and rage is tied up with your notion of mother-hood. You already hate the mother within you. *Every woman has fear about whether she will make a good mother.* You haven't given yourself permission to be a mother. You needed to clear that out. The anger and the fear are not conducive to getting pregnant."

I looked at him quizzically, struggling with what he was saying, resisting his theory. So Chris tried again, taking a more straightforward approach. "You're already doing great. But, I'm pushing you to be the best mother you can be. If, you're open to learning about your unconscious habits before you have a baby, why not do it? And these thoughts are not conducive to you becoming a mother. Now that you've let go of the physical con-tractions surrounding those thoughts and feelings, you have a good chance to resolve those feelings once and for all.

"Your job now is to stay calm," Chris urged. "Don't get pissed off. Keep life relatively simple and carefree, so you don't build up this charge again."

I initially bristled at the suggestion that I was not already liv-ing a carefree, simple life, but I had also just acknowledged, on the heels of the retreat and coming back my busy life, that I always felt like I had more to do. What's more, I often berated myself for not doing something well enough, or for taking time to relax. I approached most things in life with a certain intensity, and thus far my pregnancy project had been no different. I made a note to myself to look at how I might be able to approach conception more casually, but I felt confused as to how to do that. This felt like the most important thing I had ever undertaken, and it looked like it was going to take conscious effort to make it happen. How could I approach such a detail-oriented, high-stakes process with a care-free and casual attitude?

After Chris left, I felt shaken, stunned by the images I had seen, and humbled that I harbored these evil thoughts within me at all. Yet I was excited and open to see how this powerful session might shift my ability to get pregnant. I did feel lighter, and when I thought of my mother, I felt deep gratitude and love toward her. If nothing else, experiencing so much love for her felt amazing.

happiness despite the outcome

*A*fter my failed pregnancy attempt in June, I started to reassess my plan. Though it would mean missing my next IUI cycle, I was still intent on attending Zhixing's three-week Qigong workshop in England. Qigong blends many philosophies and ancient practices, but it has strong roots in Taoism, martial arts, and Chinese medicine. Taoists, unlike Buddhists, are obsessed with health. While Buddhists believe the body simply causes suffering, Taoists are interested in living life to the fullest potential, with the goal of cultivating the life force till the very end. Many Taoist masters, like Zhixing, live to be over one hundred years old and cultivate mythical powers. I had first studied with Zhixing in November of 2009, and had returned in August 2010 and 2011, drawn by his profound teaching and healing abilities.

Again I was putting hope into one of my masters, imagining that Zhixing might be able to improve the quality of my eggs. Though I felt cautious after asking Jamnian for help, asking Zhixing seemed different, because his work focused specifically on healing people. In the years I'd been studying with him, I had witnessed and heard many incredible stories of him successfully treating a woman for breast cancer and helping a woman, wheelchair-bound from chronic fatigue syndrome and fibromyalgia, get up out of her chair, never to return. When I asked Chris what he thought, he was enthusiastic. "If anyone can perform a miracle and help you get pregnant, it's Zhixing. He is one of the most accomplished Qigong masters I've ever seen." So in late July, I boarded a plane for England, looking forward to three gloriously long weeks of Qigong practice.

As soon as I saw Zhixing, I was struck by reverence and love for him. Greeting him always felt like a homecoming. Of all the teachers I had visited throughout the years, I felt the most synergy with and affinity to him. Although he seemed shy and barely engaged in conversation, his devotion to the practice and his students was palpable. Zhixing appeared to be weightless, ageless, and deeply grounded. While teaching, he always wore a well-tailored Chinese smock that typified my image of a Chinese master. With each step, he dropped precisely through the support of his skeleton, making him appear effortless and graceful, almost as if he was floating across the floor.

The retreat was held at a boys' boarding school in Sussex, England, on hundreds of acres of land grazed by horses and sheep. Unlike my last retreat, here I could walk the beautiful grounds, and I basked in the luxury of a dorm room all to myself. Better yet, my room was across the hall from Chris, so we often ran into each other in the hallway. I was mindful of giving Chris his space to practice, to be on this retreat as a fellow student. But I knew that he was keeping an eye on me as his student, and I felt blessed once again by his guidance and dedication.

Before my first retreat with Zhixing, Chris had warned me about the pace—short practice times and frequent tea breaks. He reassured me, "You don't need much. Trust me. Use the free time to make the practice your own." True to form, on this retreat the pace of practice appeared deceptively slow and sparse. After an early breakfast, we would start practice around ten, breaking for lunch around twelve-thirty. Then we would start again around three and practice until five. What seemed like short practice times were punctuated by several tea breaks. Between sessions, we hung around drinking ever more tea, exploring the grounds, practicing on our own, or playing Qigong games like sword form. After about a week, I began to embrace the fallow times, using them to allow the practice to percolate within my mind and body. But it was still tricky for me to trust that less could be more.

The final week of retreat, we were doing something I'd never done before: *Qi* Calligraphy. Toward the end of the second week of retreat, Zhixing set up a table at the end of the practice room and pulled out an array of calligraphy brushes and paper. We waited in anticipation to learn what Zhixing had in mind for us. When the session began, Zhixing called us over to gather around the table. "I want to paint a calligraphy for each of you as a gift," he announced as he held up a big page with over fifty different Chinese characters on it such as light, fire, home, and earth. "You can choose one of these, and I will paint it for you." This was an incredible gift. Zhixing's paintings were highly revered for their healing qualities, and even prints of the same painting were very expensive to purchase. A free, personalized, original painting was unheard of.

In *Qi* Calligraphy, the painter tunes into the *Qi* and literally allows it to move the brush. The mind of the painter is not involved in what will appear on the page. Zhixing also used the process of painting a calligraphy to treat someone. To do so, he would tune into the person and their *Qi* and then paint what he sensed— usually that on some level the *Qi* is dispersed and not contained within the body. He then encouraged the *Qi* to return to the body and condense, forcing out the smoky, stale *Qi*. This in turn would attract the *Shen* back into the body, causing deep transformation and healing. All the while, Zhixing would continue to both represent and encourage the transformation by painting the changes happening or needing to happen.

Faced with the task of choosing my own calligraphy, I felt a panic shivering on my horizon. I bought into my own superstition, creating a false truth, even though part of me knew better. *This calligraphy would have immense powers,* I told myself, *if I pick the right one.* Get it right, and I'd have a baby. Get it wrong? My chances of conception would be thwarted. No pressure, right?

As Zhixing started painting, all the students huddled around in anticipation. Initially, there was some apprehension as people contemplated what symbol they would request. A few people decided quickly, calling out a symbol that he promptly painted. Meanwhile, my self-doubt and criticism started gaining traction, picking up momentum. *Why does everyone else have the ability to pick the correct one except me? What's wrong with me?* Soon I became convinced that whatever was responsible for my lack of wisdom was also the thing that had prevented me from conceiving. In other words, I was about to fall headlong into a sea of self-judgement, but watching Zhixing paint grounded me. I could feel the strokes as they hit the paper, as if they were being painted in my body. Zhixing brought the paint brush down in a decisive thrust to make a single dot, quickly pulling the brush back up into the air. As he did so, I felt the center of my dantien light up, like he was reaching into my belly and hitting a gong located deep within. When he painted long strokes, I felt them pulling through the center of me. I was mesmerized by this symphony in my body.

My rapt attention was interrupted when a student suddenly asked for a symbol that wasn't on the chart. The resulting painting immediately inspired awe in all the students. This changed the playing field completely, as every symbol or idea under the sun became a possibility. There was a lull in student requests while people contemplated a new, bigger landscape of possibilities. In this moment, Zhixing started the next painting without a request, meaning it would be simply up for grabs. People started claiming the calligraphies even before the last stroke was formed on the page. The tension mounted. Then Maria, a sweetheart but also a hot-blooded Greek woman who often ruffled feathers amongst the rule-abiding British students, called out a claim on a calligraphy. "Oh, yes. I want that one." Then a few paintings later, she changed her mind. "No, no, I changed my mind. I want that one." Sensing impending chaos, Zhixing quickly set a ground rule, "Once you choose one, you can't change your mind. Make sure you pick the one you want!" Zhixing warned.

With this, my self-doubt exploded. I had to get this right! I contemplated a few calligraphies but didn't commit to any—how could I choose one when I didn't know what was coming next and the possibilities were endless? I started analyzing the meaning of the various calligraphies. Which would help me more—a symbol for light, home, or essence? With well over fifty people on retreat, Zhixing had many to paint. Slowly some people lost interest and the crowd started to disperse. Even as people retreated to bed, Zhixing kept painting. When I finally pulled myself away, around 10:00 P.M., I was filled with anxiety about my choice. I tossed and turned all night long, worrying about not picking the right calligraphy. When I finally fell asleep, I dreamed of calligraphies being painted. My body became the canvas and the brushstrokes washed over me all night long. When I woke up, I felt like my entire body and being were glistening from having a treatment from Zhixing throughout the night. Yet the anxiety was ever-present.

As I walked from breakfast to the practice hall, I ran into Chris. I could barely exchange a polite good morning before I launched into my concerns. "I am so anxious about picking the correct calligraphy. I'm killing myself with worry."

"Ha ha. This is good," Chris remarked. He paused for a second before continuing. "What would happen if you got the wrong calligraphy?"

I surprised myself and burst into tears as I explained, "If I don't get the right calligraphy, I'm worried that I won't get pregnant." I continued to cry, surprised at the intensity of my reaction.

"Ahh, I see. Interesting." He paused again. "Can you trust that whichever one you choose is the right one? Can you believe in the perfection of things and assume you can't do it wrong?"

"I'm just so sure I'll get it wrong," I said. Meaning, I suppose, that in that moment I could not believe in the perfection of things.

"Can you see that all of the calligraphies are an expression of love from Zhixing and thus it doesn't matter which one you get?" he continued. Then he added, jokingly, "He usually charges hundreds of dollars for a calligraphy. So it's an amazing gift no matter which one you get."

Then Chris continued on a more serious note, "What about picking a calligraphy and giving it away to someone you envy? The thing is, you are attached to the calligraphy, but you need the state, not the physical picture. Giving it away would force you to surrender your needs. It would be a selfless act. The act of a mother. A woman who wants to 'give' birth."

I paused, feeling intense pain at the thought of giving away something I perceived to be so valuable. While I could see the potential for incredible transformation in the act Chris was suggesting, I wasn't ready to give away the precious calligraphy that I still saw as holding the key to my fertility. I was gripped by desperation and a familiar self-doubt devoid of any wisdom, currently amplified by my fraught pregnancy attempts. I shifted my eyes to the floor, feeling pushed beyond my comfort zone, as I explained to Chris that I really wanted to keep the calligraphy.

"That's okay. It's a tall order, but it's something to think about in the future. The seeds have been laid. And, in the meantime, you can still untangle a lot of stuff in this. Stay grounded in the part of you that still has clarity and ponder what the underlying emotion is behind the belief that you won't get it right," Chris advised.

As soon as we said our good-byes, I walked into the practice hall to see all the calligraphies, which were now laid out on the ground on display. Some were claimed and others were still up for grabs. I immediately felt my insides lurch, and I was overcome by emotion. I rushed out of the room as tears started to fall. I was too embarrassed to let anyone see me.

I spent the next several hours trying to understand more about why I was coming undone over choosing the right calligraphy. Memories of other similar occasions flooded my mind—times when I feared I wasn't going to get or to be "enough." On Qigong retreat, I always worried about getting in enough practice. Whenever Chris asked if we wanted a break, I would always say no, worried that we needed more practice, even when I was exhausted. Similarly, on retreats, whenever rooms were not preassigned, I worried about getting a good room or a good bed. At clothing trades, I would amass huge piles of clothes in hopes of getting something good, only putting things back after trying them on. And, if in doubt, I erred on the side of keeping them. I could even see an element of this scarcity mentality in the way I used cosmetic and beauty products. I had tons of products, but I rarely finished them, fearful that I wouldn't have the product available when I needed it most. My bathroom vanity was jam packed with near-empty vials, tubes, and bottles just waiting to be finished.

This pattern was ironic in many ways, because I also knew myself to be very generous. I love to cook elaborate meals for people and give beautiful gifts. I give away clothes and food all the time. But if I looked deeply and honestly, I could also see the small hiccoughs that happened when I thought about someone else getting "better" than I had. On some level, I feared there would never be enough for me—that somehow I'd get cut out. This scarcity-mode I'd absorbed from my mother, who had grown up during World War II and the Depression. As a result of her upbringing, my mother practically never threw anything away. We had drawers filled with old wrapping paper, washed aluminum foil, quilts, and blankets. The pantry contained expired bottles of sauces and oils my mother didn't want to throw out, despite the dates stamped on their labels. She wasn't a hoarder, but she did err on the side of keeping rather than throwing things away. When I got painfully honest with myself, I could see I'd inherited the impulse to grab, to make sure I got my due, but I also felt paralyzed by the choice, the need to get it right.

I wandered the retreat grounds, wondering, *How are the inability to choose the correct calligraphy and the scarcity feeling related?* Then it dawned on me: I never felt like I was good enough, which left me feeling incomplete. I was continually seeking the panacea that would render me whole, lovable, complete: the right beauty product at the right time; the perfect outfit; more Qigong practice; or, in this case, the right calligraphy. It was all making sense.

I rushed back to the dorms, eager to share my insights with Chris before the afternoon session started. When I found him, my voice trembled as I blurted out, "I feel desperation and greediness because I want to fix myself, but my worst fear is that I might not be capable of even doing that, because I'm not good enough to figure out how to fix myself." I continued, working hard to get the words out as emotion swept over me, "The perfection of things you spoke of is unfathomable." I confessed. "Even if it exists, I don't believe it could apply to *me*. I'm too flawed. I'm too inadequate to pick the right calligraphy. Thus, a feeling of grasping takes over."

I could sense Chris trying to understand my visceral experience, to fully grasp it above and beyond my words. I saw him scanning my system before he responded, "I know it feels painful. Everyone thinks they are fundamentally flawed in some way. The practice is to notice your perfection. You can't do it wrong," he said tenderly. "The good news is that you are on the right track. Try to boil down all these ideas and sensations into one word or feeling," he urged. "Can you see all those behaviors as one thing? Don't be too clever. Try to simplify."

I pondered some more. I felt like I was taxing my brain in an effort to think harder and figure it out. "It feels like desperation, but I guess there's a greediness in it too."

Chris proceeded cautiously, "Yes. If I were to give it a name, I'd call it the 'gimmes.' It's like a sensation of 'Give me that' or 'This is mine.' Can you feel that?" He paused to let his words sink in. "When you sense that feeling arise, recognize that you are feeling inadequate. Label it the 'gimmes' feeling and stop it. It's based on old software. It's why you can't contemplate giving away your calligraphy, but it's not who you really are at your essence."

Suddenly, something locked into place for me. "Yes, I can feel that. I'm still not sure how to untie it from not feeling good enough, but it does make sense."

"You might not be able to solve not feeling good enough right away, but you can get familiar with the 'gimme' tendency, develop a bandwidth to tolerate it, and decide not to indulge it. And, by softening the somatic sensation that goes along with it, you can untie the tendency for good." Chris was explaining the familiar process of naming and mapping something so that I could more easily recognize it and let it go. Rather than unconsciously being caught in its grip and blindly following the mind stream of information, I could shine a light of awareness upon it. "This desperation and greediness would be good to clean up, especially before you have a child. It would be great if you didn't teach it to your child." Here it was again—the invitation to look deeply into my mental baggage so that I could have as clean an environment as possible in which to welcome my future child. This never-ending learning—it's what called me to Qigong and life coaching—I continually wanted to refine my motivations and mental habits. If I had never learned how to look inside, I'd still be blissfully ignorant to much of this. But I'd committed to living as consciously as possible, so here I was looking at ingrained habits and releasing them, yet again.

While I continued to be triggered when I thought about picking the "right" calligraphy, tumbling into a cascade of mental haranguing, I had taken in the mental lesson. I worked to release my body from the grip, training myself to remain centered in the face of the unpleasant message. Rather than being overcome by it, I could learn to hear it in the background. Slowly I would desensitize myself, loosening my visceral response to the "gimmes," by exposing myself to the triggering source repeatedly. Each time I saw the calligraphies or thought about picking one, I noticed myself get thrown off center, and I carefully found my bones and breath again, recovering in the moment. Eventually my initial response scaled down, and I was able to get back home more quickly.

The next morning, I walked through the room where all the unclaimed calligraphies lay, one of them jumped out at me. I picked it up off the ground, called by it like no other. Zhixing was standing close by, so I asked him what it meant. "It's enjoyment!" he exclaimed. "But more importantly, it's enjoyment and happiness no matter what the outcome—no matter the external circumstances. It's a very Taoist form of enjoyment—the happiness that comes from within."

I almost fell over laughing. How much more perfect could it be? Here I was, holding the key to my liberation—happiness no matter what the outcome. Happiness regardless of whether or not I could get pregnant or find a partner; contentment no matter which calligraphy I received. How happy and simple would life be if I could adopt this philosophy? Maybe I would even eventually trust the perfection of this rollercoaster journey to pregnancy? I committed to the calligraphy on the spot, my incessant internal dialogue silenced.

Over the next few days, Zhixing's new calligraphies seemed to take on lives of their own, getting more and more artistic. As they appeared, if I noticed a pang of regret, I quickly reminded myself, "happiness no matter what the outcome." Each time, I affirmed the perfection of my choice.

On August 23, the last day of the retreat, I visited the toilet before the long car journey to the airport. I was elated to see that I had started my period, the first one since my failed insemination attempt in June. It seemed like a good omen, starting a new cycle as I returned to the US, freshly charged up from my three-week retreat. Maybe I could actually get pregnant this time?

As I said good-bye to Chris, who was off to visit friends in London, he shared some parting words. "Just relax. Keep it simple. Try not to get upset. Remember that your entire nervous system is on a hair trigger. The slightest negative thought destabilizes your chemistry. You need everything in your system to work toward making the happy, healthy hormones to conceive a child. So, try to calm down your mind and your body. Keep life easy. Settle your system down. And, more than anything, believe that you can do this."

This little pep talk reminded me of all the times Chris had told me that my nervous system would love to live in a monastery. "The level of stimulus in a monastery is about as much input as your system can handle," he'd tell me. "You're like the most delicate leaf. The slightest puff of air sends you twirling off the branch to the ground."

Though "relax" seemed a simple enough instruction, it could be one of the hardest things to do. The desire to get things done always seemed to win out. As I sat on the plane from Heathrow to San Francisco, I pulled out my journal and made some commitments to myself. I would practice Qigong every day and keep life simple. I would notice and avoid all the distractions and seemingly urgent tasks. I would start everything I did with a question to myself, "Is this really urgent right now?" Slow and simple—that was my new life motto (at least for a few months). With these promises made, I felt charged up, healthy, and hopeful.

As soon as I got home, I started tracking. I juggled morning body temperature, saliva monitor, and daily pee sticks from several different ovulation predictor kits. I felt my cervix, noted cervical fluid—you name it, I did it. I tried to approach the ceaseless tracking with the blissful, happy mind I'd cultivated on retreat, but I won't lie: when scurrying to catch every last ambiguous symptom, it was hard to maintain a light mind. I knew that the mind with which I'd been approaching my fertility journey thus far was likely getting in the way of my miracle, so I tried in earnest to shift it. As a result, I managed to live a relatively calm few weeks. I spent my days walking my dogs, eating healthy food, doing my Qigong practice morning and night, while seeing a handful of clients and teaching my Qigong classes. I laid in the sun and rested, keeping life as simple and unemotional as possible.

Meanwhile, things were beginning to line up in my favor. By day ten, my saliva showed a partial ferning pattern indicating an estrogen spike. On day twelve, I got positive OPKs on two out of three of the three different brands I was neurotically monitoring. I called Michelle, who arrived around 11:00 P.M. to do the first IUI, but my cervix was not open enough. We both felt confident that we were still too early, so we scheduled the next attempt for six o'clock the following morning with Rebecca.

When I woke up on Sunday, day thirteen, I was thrilled to see that my cervical fluid was the consistency of egg whites—something I had rarely seen before—and my cervix felt soft and open. My excitement grew. When Rebecca arrived, the catheter passed through my cervix, though I felt a pinch of pain. Rebecca assured me that could happen, and it didn't lower my chances of conceiving. Michelle returned on Monday morning, day fourteen, at six, for the second IUI, and the catheter again easily passed through my cervix. I lay in bed after the IUI, fervently saying mantras and listening to meditation recordings by Zhixing. I invited in a baby spirit and prayed for success. I put every ounce of my being into this effort. By 10:00 P.M., I could feel that my cervix felt hard and closed, and my excitement mounted. My body had exhibited a much clearer pattern than ever before, and it appeared that we had timed the IUIs perfectly. When I woke up Tuesday, I was even more thrilled to see that my temperature had indeed spiked. When I went to the bathroom, however, I noticed faint spotting. I put in a panty liner, telling myself that it was because of the first IUI when Rebecca had to push the catheter a bit to pass through my cervix.

As I taught my Qigong class that morning, I was elated. My students remarked at how happy and buoyant I seemed.

"You're positively glowing," one of my regular students remarked.

I was dying to tell them, but I decided it was too risky. "I'm just really happy today," I responded. "I don't know why." Though, of course, I knew exactly why. As I got in my car to drive home, however, I felt a big gush in my pants, and when I got home, I saw that I had soaked through a panty liner with blood and what felt like other fluid. *It must have been bleeding from the IUI, right?* Though this theory didn't account for the other fluids I thought I'd felt. I called Michelle, who agreed that it was possible the bleeding was caused by the IUI, though we were both confused by my description of other fluids. I switched tracks. *Maybe instead it was implantation bleeding?* A quick Google search explained that implantation bleeding usually occurs about seven to ten days after fertilization when the embryo implants itself into the uterine wall. However, some women report bleeding as early as five days after ovulation. Definitely a far-fetched theory, but another testament to how crazy hope and uncertainty can make a person.

The next morning, my temperature had spiked even more dramatically, and that day I felt the same pain I regularly associated with ovulation on the left side of my pelvis. Even though I was cautious, I still believed that everything was looking good. On day eighteen, however, my temperature, which had continued to climb, dropped dramatically. I hoped it was simply a bad reading, but for the next few days it continued to drop and the erratic bleeding continued. But I was not giving up hope yet! I was convinced that the combination of the retreat with Zhixing and what appeared to be a very clear pattern of bodily symptoms leading up to ovulation was the magic combination. I was determined to hold out hope for a few more days.

In hindsight, I see the improbability, and I wonder where my sane and reasonable self was hiding? But hope turns reason on its head sometimes. In the thick of my journey, I happily interpreted any ambiguity in favor of a positive outcome. I fixated on the outcome—a positive outcome, specifically—rather than accepting the uncertainty of trying to conceive. Ultimately, that need to predict an outcome, that unwillingness to let the unknown simply be unknown, even in the midst of wildly ambiguous symptoms, caused so much suffering. From what I've read on message boards, this seems a common reaction to the dreaded two-week wait.

The ambiguity disappeared on day twenty-five. I was walking my dogs when I experienced a sharp pain on the right side of my pelvis. It was so bad that I doubled over, unable to walk for a few minutes. Later that day, I began bleeding heavily. Why I had been bleeding on and off since presumed ovulation remained a mystery, but the question of whether I was pregnant had been unequivocally answered.

I fell hard, as if a giant black hole opened up and swallowed me, cold and dark and filled with despair. I was sure this cycle was going to be the *one.* I turned off my phone, unable to bear any contact with the outside world. I curled up into the safety of my bed, trying not to think about the $2000 I'd just spent on sperm vials and insemination fees, and I started to cry. Neither of the two previous failed inseminations hit me as hard as this one. I was beginning to lose hope.

ending self-hatred:
doing the best i can

*I*n early July, before I left for England, I had finally scheduled an appointment with a reproductive endocrinologist to run some more tests and get her opinion about my
chances of getting pregnant. She'd run my AMH (anti-mullerian
hormone) and resting follicle count, as well as rerunning my FSH.
She explained that the three measures taken together were predic-
tive of egg quality and quantity. As it turned out, my FSH had gone
up slightly to 25.4, I had only one resting follicle on each ovary (a
woman in the peak of her fertility might have up to twenty per
ovary), and my AMH was undetectable. With these numbers, not
only did she not recommend IVF, but said she would refuse to treat
me with IVF even if I wanted to try it. At the time, I had brushed
these numbers out of my psyche, not wanting to allow them
to deter my confidence. But now, a month after the third failed
insemination attempt and with ever more erratic periods, the reality of those numbers hit me. Luckily, around this same time, Chris
was offering a Qigong retreat. A chance to get away from my life to
do Qigong practice all day long? I took it.

The retreat center was in Calistoga, just north of the Bay
Area, with stunning views of the surrounding wine country and

mountains, with acres of walking trails to explore. As soon as I arrived at the center, I stopped to take in nature's beauty. In an effort to arrive more fully, I took a deep breath, linking to nature and welcoming the influence of the qualities present. My body opened to the expansiveness of the view. I carried this feeling into the practice hall, joining about twenty other students in a circle. I sat on my chair, my back was easily upright, my feet on the floor shoulder-width apart, my hands gently clasped in my lap. The sun streamed through the French doors lining the wall, drenching my body in its warmth. I glanced out the windows into the garden teeming with vegetables and fruits ready for harvest.

Chris wasn't a big fan of long, drawn out check-ins or intro-ductions, so with this retreat he had decided to jump right in. "Let's start by paying attention to the breathing," he began. "Try not to concoct the breath in any way, but instead just listen. Simply notice all the places that the body moves with the breath." I fol-lowed his instruction, melting into the peace of the practice. As I'd been trained, I turned my attention to noticing how the pressure of the breath affected every part of the body. I scanned the body, looking for new and interesting places that my breath was moving my body: the small of my low back, my shoulder blades moving in and out across my ribs, my arms lifting up and down. As my mind slowed down, and I became more and more present to my current experience. I could even perceive my feet moving a tiny bit with each breath.

A few minutes into the practice, Chris gave us more detail. "There's a space between the tip of the shoulder and the neck. It lies between the clavicle and the shoulder blade in the back. If you put your fingers there, you can feel a soft spot—a little space." He paused to give us time to sense and feel what he was talking about. "The lungs reach all the way up to this space. Listen to this space in more detail." As I tuned into this area, I started to see my breath in glorious Technicolor, as I perceived bigger and bigger movements up and down, giving way to images. I was struck with awe as I marveled at the perfection of the body. Had I noticed the move-ment in this area before now? My neck and clavicle made the shape of a metal coat hanger, my clavicle forming the bottom, my neck the sloping sides. With each breath, the clavicle rose and fell, causing the sides of the hanger to rise and fall, as if collapsing in on itself and then expanding. If one part moved, all parts moved. I sat for several minutes, watching this movement, completely absorbed in the observation.

Then, out of nowhere, a thought arose. *I never really get it.* My mood deflated, and I started to wonder what other people were experiencing. *What I'm noticing is so inferior to what other people notice, and I never understand meditation.* At first, I let these thoughts float by, trying not to grasp at them, just observing them as they moved through me. I'd met thoughts like these many times before—comparing, assuming I'm not enough. Because I was so familiar with this pattern, I had learned to see it as a trap. Chris often described this type of thinking as faulty output from a computer, because these thoughts are largely learned and not part of one's essence. The trick was simply to delete the faulty output and move on without giving power to or believing the thoughts. Some days, deleting the output was easier to accomplish than others. On this day, I couldn't stop myself from falling down the rabbit hole of self-hatred.

As the day wore on, the thoughts worsened. I continued comparing myself to other people on the retreat. I knew this was poison, but I couldn't stop myself. By the end of the day, I had convinced myself I did not understand anything about Qigong at all. In fact, I had no right to teach Qigong. Before long, my thoughts generalized to my entire being—I was a fraud and a terrible person too. I was spiraling out of control. I was tethered to clarity just enough to know it was time to ask Chris for help, so I found him during one of the breaks by the tea station. I leaned against a table feeling completely deflated and unable to stand without support. "Why don't I ever understand Qigong?" I asked slumping even further as I thought about my inadequacies. "I'm so bad at it. Why do other people understand it so much better than me?"

Rather than feeding into my spiraling thoughts, Chris responded by asking, "Let me ask you this: Why do you practice?

Can you connect to that reason?" He continued, "If you can connect to this deeper calling, you can relax about the techniques. Whether or not you 'get it' becomes irrelevant."

"I guess so," I responded. In the past, when I had pondered this question, I discovered that I practiced in order to live a conscious life. I wanted continually to shine a light of awareness onto myself, and by doing so, I hoped to live in accordance with my true nature. Further, I taught Qigong because I wanted to share the beauty and clarity I had discovered through the practice. But at the moment, tangled in self-doubt, those seemed like distant reasons. The tea break was over, so I forced myself to return to the practice room and sit down.

Chris began, "Many people have come to me with questions that I think I can answer in the group. Let me ask you this: why do you practice?"

A student raised her hand, "I'm confused. Can you give us an example?"

"Sure. Many people, when they first start to practice, do so because they are sick or have a health or emotional issue they are working on. But at a certain point, they fix the problem. They don't need to practice anymore to fix that problem. But they still do. At other times, people decide to give up the practice for some reason or another. But before too long, they return because something deeper calls them back to practice. For me, it's devotion. When I remember my devotion, I have no other choice but to practice. Just as I have no choice whether or not to breathe. This calls me back to the meaning and real reason for my practice. It's no longer a question. And it no longer matters if I'm bad or good at it."

Yeah, yeah, I thought. *That's all really nice, but for the last few months I've been practicing because I view it as my only hope for getting pregnant. I've thrown myself more deeply into my practice than any other time in my life, and where has that gotten me?* In this desperate moment, I needed to *get* Qigong, needed to be *good* at it, or I'd never have a baby. The idea of a higher calling or greater purpose seemed quaint, completely irrelevant in light of my urgent project. Thoughts about my three failed inseminations buzzed in my brain, and I started to panic. Then I recalled Chris' advice, "Give it your best shot. Figure out what you need to do in order to feel like you did the best you could. That way, you can be at peace if you have to move on to something else."

Every time Chris had said this to me, I felt my whole system recoil in disbelief. I felt completely incapable of doing a good enough job. I would beat myself up for all my small missteps, like not practicing every day or not practicing for long enough. I'd remember how many times I'd I had a glass of wine, eaten dairy, or stayed out late. I convinced myself that these transgressions were enough to throw off the delicate balance I was trying to cultivate. And now, as I listened to Chris repeat this familiar soundtrack, my despair began gaining steam. *I could have done a much better job at trying to get pregnant. And why did I wait so dammed long to decide to have a baby alone?* As I raged on in my head, Chris started to lead us through a meditation to help us connect to the deeper reasons we practiced. He directed our attention back to our breathing. "Tell yourself not to breathe. Can you do it?" he asked. "Tell yourself not to digest your food. Again, you can't do it. Your body is tirelessly working, and you can't make it stop."

Chris's voice gave me a break from my thoughts, and again I sunk into my body, marveling at its unending service to me. *The body truly is a marvelous miracle.* But in practically the same breath, I tapped into a reservoir of rage against my reproductive system for not working properly. My body wasn't miraculous, because it was failing me now when I wanted to have a baby. Why had I waited so long? Why hadn't I been able to find a partner and been able to have a baby when I was younger and more fertile? What was wrong with my body? Why didn't I do more fertility tests earlier and realize how little time I had? Why didn't I practice Qigong and meditation more diligently so I could fix myself? The thoughts went on and on, gaining momentum like an avalanche tumbling down a mountainside.

When the meditation ended, I sat stunned by the depth of this anger and self-loathing. But the scarier part was that the stream of thoughts was so familiar. I was not only desperately angry at myself in this moment, but I'd been living under constant attack, ever since I had decided to have a baby on my own. These voices of disapproval and anger were constant. Sometimes they lurked under the radar, barely audible. Other times they were loud and obvious, but regardless, they were vicious, harsh, and unrelenting, whether I consciously realized them or not.

When Chris directed us to stand so we could continue our exploration, these feelings stood with me. He directed us to raise our arms to perform the standing prostration exercise used to condense the *Qi* around the body. It was a familiar, flowing pattern I'd done thousands of times before. But as I moved my arms, I was distracted by the rage that had unleashed. I felt physically heavy, unable to find the energy to hold up my arms. The simplest movement felt like drawing my arms through hardening concrete. Completely defeated, I dropped to my knees and curled up into a ball on the floor. After a few moments, I managed to pull myself up from the floor and raised my arms, in an attempt to stay with the practice. But inevitably, I started to cry and curled back up into a ball on the ground. It's not unusual for people to have strong emotional experiences on retreat, so no one moved toward me. People gave me space and trusted that I would be okay eventually. I wish I could have said the same for myself. For the rest of the day, my mood persisted. At meals, I kept my head down and refused to connect with my fellow students.

It was unlike me to leave the practice room or stop practicing. No matter how bad it got, I trusted the practice and believed that I could work through my emotions by staying present. I looked forward to the insight that I knew would come eventually if I was willing to face whatever difficulty was arising. But the next morning, I had arrived at the practice session still unable to break out of my funk and I felt unable to do the practice. My body seemed incapable of following the movements. Defeated, I went outside to sit on bench on the deck attached to the practice room. I was hoping the sun and beauty of my surroundings would help snap me out of it. But I continued to cry. With intention, I could put things into perspective, but only for moments at a time before awful thoughts of what a shameful person I was would flood my system, and I'd start to cry again.

After well over an hour, Chris came out to the deck to check on me. "I feel so helpless. I can see and feel the self-hatred coursing through my body," I explained. "There's a part of my mind that sees that I am unfairly torturing myself and has enough reason to feel compassionate and forgiving about how I ended up single and potentially infertile. But the hatred keeps winning out, popping its head out from behind the shadows telling me how horrible I am." As I spoke, a wave of anger washed through me. "I don't know how to get out of this. The pain feels never-ending."

Chris nodded reassuringly and sat with me for a while as I sobbed. "I know it doesn't feel like it," he ventured, "but you're actually doing great. But you need to keep going. As scary as it seems, I would completely indulge in your story and negative thoughts. It's rare that people have the courage to look directly at the negativity—they run away from it so it never fully gets processed. But I know you can handle it. I don't think it will take long to get to the bottom of the well."

"This is great?" I asked in disbelief.

"Yes," he reassured me, placing his hand on my shoulder and looking me in the eye warmly. "You've been practicing long enough to find your way through this." Although my current state of mind made it difficult to believe I was capable of anything good, I knew that Chris was directing me to follow a Taoist progression. Rather than shying away from the feelings and experience, he was encouraging me to follow it to its furthest point. Only then would the pendulum swing back the other way and eventually reach equilibrium.

I spent the rest of the morning session outside, but after our lunch break I ventured back into the room. As we sat in a circle, checking in about how things were going, a newer student said to the group and to me, "Sarah, I want to recognize that I see you are in pain. Please let me know if I can help you." I nodded and tried to smile in recognition, but was unable to speak. It was clear that she was questioning Chris's hands-off approach.

He responded, "When someone is going through a process, I am always watching and keeping track. I won't let someone go farther than they can handle. And even if I'm not right by the person's side, I know what's going on, and I'm monitoring their process. Class is always happening on many levels, and I have my eye on several different people all at once, even though I'm not in physical proximity to them. So, don't worry, everyone in the room is getting what they need."

I knew this to be true. I'd been in enough retreats with Chris and had struggled through many difficult times under his care. Still, it was good to hear again as I grappled with this uncomfortable set of thoughts and emotions.

The final morning of retreat, we gathered in the practice room, and Chris led us through the progression we'd been practicing all week. I was still resistant to being in the room, but I knew I needed to stay to work through my funk, in hopes of popping out the other side. For most of the week, I'd felt weak and unable to practice. But now, I started to feel currents of sensation mounting in my system. Emotions would come rushing to the surface, and I'd begin to cry again, but the sadness quickly transformed into anger. The now familiar soundtrack about my body's inability to perform the basic functions of a woman started to gain force. I let the force grow, trusting I would blow through to the other side eventually. Overcome with rage at my ovaries and reproductive system, I allowed a scream to erupt, piercing the air with its force. Cognizant of the other students in the room, I wanted to stop the sound, but the intensity was too much to bear—I had to give it voice. I gave myself permission to continue, knowing the other students would understand the release.

The force of anger traveling through my body pushed me onto the ground, near a blanket that had been left at the edge of the room. As the mounting rage urged me to rip my hair out in clumps or claw my skin off, I crouched on the blanket, gripping it until my knuckles turned white, giving my hands something to do as a scream arose again, voicing the self-destructive energy. As the sound unleashed, I was vaguely aware of some children perched on stairs on the deck just outside the open French doors. Where did they come from? What in the world they were doing there, at this very moment? Chris calmly walked over and closed the doors, creating a barrier between my screams and the children sitting outside. Even though he did not demonstrate that he was in any way upset, I immediately took his actions as a comment on my behavior and started berating myself for making too much noise. Nevertheless, I continued to scream and cry, battling waves of self-destructive rage.

I have no idea how long this went on. I was aware that I must be disturbing the other students, but Chris had essentially trained us to respect and allow everyone's experience, from hysterical laughing attacks to anger and rage. This, however, seemed larger and more dramatic than anyone's experience in a long time. But I could not pull myself back, and I knew I needed to go through this rage in order to come out the other side. After what may have been twenty to thirty minutes, according to what some students told me afterward, I was suddenly hit with a more intense urge to hurt myself. I was convinced I could no longer hold myself back. I screamed for help. "Help me, Chris! Help me! I'm going to hurt myself!" I screamed. "I want to rip out my hair or scratch off my skin, and I don't think I can stop myself!"

Chris stood in front of me, pointing his fingers toward the ground in a gesture that I knew was to help me ground myself and stop the reaction I was having. At first there was a rather intense crescendo, but I quickly came to a relative peace and gained more conscious control of my mind. "How are you doing now?" he asked.

"I still have an urge to pull out my hair. It's a deeply visceral desire, but I know I can control myself," I said, still kneeling on the floor, gripping the blanket and heaving to get air.

Now the entire room of students was watching me, and I could feel their concern. It's rare for anyone to call for support. Chris must have also sensed that people were too distracted and concerned to practice, so he called for a break.

When he turned back to me, I continued, "I'm shocked at the intensity of the hateful thoughts I have toward myself. They were strong enough to make me want to destroy myself for being such a terrible person. I can't believe I function on a day-to-day basis with these demons living internally."

Chris nodded reassuringly as he came to sit next to me on the ground. "This is good to see. This will motivate you to stop this destructive line of thought. But you also need to realize that this is something that was passed on to you through your family line. The anger you feel about not being able to conceive is stirring up these feelings that normally lay relatively dormant below your conscious awareness. So although it's deeply ingrained and learned, you can also escape it very easily."

He sat with me a bit longer as I continued to calm down, then he called the class back together, inviting us to pull out chairs and sit in a circle. We often debriefed the sessions afterward, and this one definitely needed some discussion. Some of the students, especially newer ones who weren't accustomed to the chaotic aspects of class, must have been pretty freaked out by the experience, especially my sudden plea for help. Chris offered an opportunity for the class to share thoughts or ask questions.

My friend and long-time fellow Qigong student, Genevieve, raised her hand sheepishly. She began with a preface of sorts. She looked at me apologetically as she spoke. "I'm sorry, Sarah. I hope this doesn't upset you, but I want to understand my own experience." I nodded to let her know it was okay to continue. I knew that she would not in any way try to hurt me or offend me. She continued with a beaming smile on her face. "That was one of the most beautiful experiences I have ever had. If I ever doubted the existence of God, I now know with certainty that there is a God," she explained. "As Sarah sunk deeper and deeper into despair and darkness, I could perceive something that kept getting brighter and more beautiful. It was the brightest, purest, most beautiful light I have ever seen. And there was a perfection in all aspects, even the children who were perched on the steps. It was like they were all part of the plan to balance out the pain and darkness. It was like an equal and opposite force was coming to meet her pain. As her suffering grew worse, the light came to balance it."

Chris nodded in agreement. "Yes," he said, "as Sarah cried in pain, it was like a prayer. The sincerity of the cry for help and the depth of the pain summoned immense help. Her prayer was answered even though she may not realize it yet. This is the meaning of Yin and Yang. As her darkness was summoned, the brightness arrived to balance it. She has help now to deal with this. You could say her prayers have been answered. She's seen through to the depth of the pain and can find a way out now."

This exchange put everyone at ease. Students moved on to asking questions about the retreat in general. Meanwhile, I tried to digest the idea of this beautiful perfection Genevieve had witnessed. To the extent that I'd been cognizant of anything while I'd been screaming on the floor, I had been worrying about bothering my fellow students. I never guessed that my pain would lead someone else to a steadfast belief in the divine. I marveled at life's irony and tried to absorb the idea of the perfection of my experience.

When the session ended, I approached Chris again, feeling largely recovered. I wanted to understand more about how to end this self-hatred once and for all. "What do I do with that experience? How do I make sure that it comes to something?"

"I really think it's done," he said. "That's why I let you go as long as I did. I could see a process taking place that I did not want to interrupt. I think the answer will appear to you."

I didn't feel so sure. The look on my face must have conveyed that because Chris continued, "You have a few options if you want to actively do something. You could recognize the standard of life without this hatred and stop tolerating any hateful thoughts. Bathe in the idea that you are doing the best you can. Spend a little time every day bathing in goodness, until it becomes your new habit. Or you could work with it somatically by trying to gain some separation between your body and the feelings. This would involve desensitizing yourself to the reaction. Practice looking in a mirror and noticing all the contractions and sensations associated with

self-hatred that arise and try to soften them. Can you work on having the thoughts with less physical response?"

I believed I could do this, and now was the time. I knew my
road to pregnancy would continue to be difficult. I needed to let
go of how mad I was at myself for not being able to conceive, or I
would destroy myself in the process.

losing faith

After returning from my retreat in mid-October, I did another IUI in early November. No go. In mid-November, I had another period, and I jumped into gear for another IUI mid-December. Once again, based on a truly embarrassing number of OPKs and cross-referenced bodily symptoms, it appeared I'd timed ovulation correctly. Once again, no go. I was beginning to wonder if I was not ovulating altogether, or if I was ovulating but something was preventing my body from producing enough progesterone to sustain a pregnancy? Nowhere in my online research could I find the answers.

Meanwhile, the engine behind Project Baby—namely, me—was definitely losing steam. I had been so diligent—practicing Qigong and meditation daily, eating the right foods, ingesting my mountain of supplements, and generally trying to relax in order to set my body up to be ready to conceive, all amounting to nothing. On the one hand, there wasn't much more I could do, and on the other, I had a constant, nagging feeling that I should be doing more. At the outset, for every IUI, I had to believe it was going to work, because I believed that my mental state influenced my chances, but that also meant that I was gutted each time a pregnancy test turned up another Big Fat Negative. Cycle after cycle, I felt like I'd been climbing an intense hill, over and over, only to tumble down to the bottom before I ever reached the top. Frankly, I was exhausted by both the repetitive hope-disappointment cycle and by the dogged diligence I had brought to Project Baby for the past ten months.

After December's negative pregnancy test, I was sick of it all. Sick of being a good girl. Sick of practicing Qigong hours every day, abstaining from alcohol, and avoiding wheat or dairy. A rebellion mounted. Of course, after a period of such austerity, rebellion looked tame—I poured myself a nice, big glass of wine and jumped in a very hot bath, which I'd been avoiding because they can negatively affect fertility. I went to bed that night without doing the Qigong and meditation practice I'd practiced every night before bed for the past six months. In the morning, I took myself out to my favorite café to get reacquainted with some old friends: gluten, sugar, dairy, and caffeine. With the purchase of a latte and a pastry, I flipped the bird at everyone in the natural fertility-boosting world, who admonished dairy and gluten so strongly you'd think they were heroin and cocaine.

The rebellion continued for several weeks. Instead of doing Qigong, I binged on episodes of *True Blood* and *Breaking Bad*. I liberated myself from supplements and herbal teas, replacing them with lattes and cappuccinos—caffeinated, with *cow's* milk, thank you very much—breaking a ten-year caffeine fast and a ten-month dairy ban. One night, I decided to have a glass of wine, and then another and another. With my wine goggles on, I developed a new mantra: "Screw it. I don't care." I yearned for a way to simply check out, to stop thinking about my fertility, or lack thereof. I had never wanted anything so badly as I wanted a baby. I had never been so focused or worked so hard in my life to attain something. But despite my greatest efforts, I was no closer to motherhood than I had been when Project Baby began.

Maybe I should take this rebellion further, I thought. My friend Laura had been inviting me to stay at her hotel in Mexico for over a year, and I kept putting it off, prioritizing pregnancy over anything else. For the last few months, I'd been thinking about visiting, but I couldn't because I couldn't predict when my period would come. In the center of this fatalistic burnout, the idea rekindled. I could dance, play, and swim in the gorgeous bathtub-temperature ocean.

But every time I started to look for tickets, I would pull myself back, knowing I needed to stay focused and in the US, where I could do an insemination whenever my body indicated it might be moving toward ovulation. While my "screw it" mantra chanted on, Chris had been traveling in India for two months. I scheduled an appointment with him as soon as he returned. Entering his treatment room, I felt like the Catholic schoolgirl I once was, headed to confession. "I am so sick of taking such good care of myself," I told him. "It doesn't seem like it's helping at all, so I've been abusing my body by drinking wine, eating gluten and dairy, staying out late, and refusing to do Qigong practice. And now I'm just sad and exhausted. I can't even begin to explain how tired I feel."

"That's good," he explained. "Follow the frustration and exhaustion. Let it flow out rather than trying to contain it or be good. Since you just spent ten months being good and doing all the right things, it's understandable that you need to rebel. Give it up and relax. If you deny your feelings, they will simply get stuffed down into the recesses of your mind and continue to wreak havoc. On the other hand, if you can give voice to your exhaustion without guilt, it will run its course and resolve much more quickly."

Though this approach felt a bit reckless, it resonated with me. I had tried a similar method in the past, when I went through a horribly lazy and tired period in my life. Instead of pushing myself to be productive amidst the laziness, I followed it completely. I sat on the couch, determined to stay as long as I wanted, not getting out of my pajamas, luxuriating in being a complete sloth. Inevitably, by the end of the second day, I was up and taking care of business. Not because I thought I should or because I was forcing myself out of guilt, but because I had rested and gotten it out of my system. Once again this Taoist principle had proven itself: by allowing the extremes to exist, I rebalanced in the middle very quickly. Now here I was again, faced with an opportunity to follow a direction completely, so it could run its course and right itself again.

"It's the guilt that's toxic," Chris explained. "It creates a host of co-contractions in the body and mind. If you can just drink or rebel in whatever way you choose without the guilt, it will be over much faster. Fully indulge rather than doing it in some half-assed way," he encouraged. Indulge the impulse *without* the guilt? In the history of Catholicism, no priest had uttered those words in a confessional. Chris was telling me to do the exact opposite of my upbringing, and it felt liberating. "Why don't you lay on the table and I'll see if I can help you with the exhaustion," he suggested.

I felt like I needed a tune-up, so I happily laid down and started to relax. Chris began waving his arms a few inches above my body in big sweeps from the middle of my torso out through my legs, using *BuQi* techniques to help remove the stale *Qi* in my system.

"Make no assumptions about whether you are being bad or good," Chris continued. "How do you know if eating wheat or drinking wine will help or hurt your efforts to get pregnant? Devalue everything and stop doing anything because you think you *should*. Consider all things equally, and then see what you are called to do," he explained with increasing fervor. "Don't assume that going to see a spiritual teacher is better for you or has more value than going to Mexico to lay in the sun and go salsa dancing. If you can stop following that which society or your internal critic thinks has value, and begin to follow what feels correct or is in your true nature, your intrinsic nature has a chance to come out."

Chris had always cautioned against certain diets or supplements as a solution, as he believed what worked for one person's system might not necessarily work for another's. He bordered on fanatical in his desire to teach his students to hone their own ability to sense what was best for their own systems. "Trust only your own internal authority," he would admonish. "The problem is that most people never pay close enough attention to understand what's working for their system. That causes them to be dependent on outside authority. But a good Qigong practitioner should be able to sense what they, as an individual, need."

A light bulb went off in my head, and suddenly I had a new perspective about how I'd been approaching pregnancy for these past ten months. Because I had strong research and knowledge-gathering skills, I'd uncovered tons of conflicting information about how to boost my fertility. I had spent months avoiding dairy at the advice of acupuncturists and naturopaths, and then a friend had sent me a study that showed women who had at least one serving of full fat dairy a day had a higher success rate in getting pregnant. After taking melatonin for a few months, I had found conflicting data about its effects. Some evidence suggested that taking melatonin could cause premature ovarian failure. Yet another study showed that women who had previously not been able to get pregnant conceived after taking melatonin for a month. I'd been tearing my hair out over these kinds of conflicts. Should I cut out dairy and wheat or not? Should I go to Mexico, or stay home living an austere life? The contradictory information was enough to make a want-to-be mama crazy. In the face of contrary advice, it was ridiculous to do anything *but* follow my own internal sensations. The idea of valuing all the choices in front of me equally, then deciding based on my internal drive—this was truly cathartic.

"You've been trying thus far, with effort and determination. You are really good at putting your mind to something and going at it with sweat and determination. In this case, you gave up many things, took all the supplements, saw many practitioners, and practiced with a certain intensity around getting pregnant. You've done the good-girl thing," Chris acknowledged, "but that path has a certain amount of anxiety and tension in it, because you've created so many rules. That anxiety could, in and of itself, be preventing you from getting pregnant. Try something different, and just follow what feels appropriate. Try without trying. Just be free."

I left my session with Chris feeling like my entire orientation had been turned upside down. While it would be difficult to unlearn my habit of tackling problems head-on, I was curious to see where this advice might lead me. I developed a new mantra: "Just follow. Don't be the good girl!" Walking through my days with this gentle, persistent reminder by my side, I started to notice how many things I did because I thought I should, or because I thought it was good for me, with no reference to my internal compass.

After a few days, while I was out walking my dogs in the nearby redwood forest, these words popped into my mind: *I did the best I could to get pregnant*. At first, I thought someone else was inhabiting my brain—this was *not* how I thought. Throughout my efforts to get pregnant, Chris had counseled me, "Do whatever it takes to feel like you did the best you could. If you can do that, you'll be able to walk away without regret, if necessary." But I had never felt I was doing my best. My internal critic was ever present, ready to call into question the diligence of my efforts, highlighting the moments when I faltered in my determination by cheating on my strict diet or failing to do my daily Qigong practice. When Chris and I had revisited the topic in late October, I scoffed at the notion that anyone feels like they did their best. I couldn't fathom that some people lived free of this relentless, internal criticism. "No truly," Chris explained, "I can look at almost any aspect of my life and say I did the best I could."

"That's just because you're practically enlightened," I scoffed. "Normal people don't feel that way. If I look at any aspect of my life and try to say, 'I did the best I could,' I am confronted by utter disbelief and repulsion."

"I think you will find that many people feel this way," Chris suggested. "Ask some of your friends and see what they say. You might be surprised."

I set to work asking my friends, "Do you ever feel like you did the best you could?" I was astonished to find out that my friends could say that, in many aspects of their lives, they had done the best they could. For me, making this claim seemed a far-off, unattainable goal. But three months later, as I stood in the depths of the forest with my dogs, I could say with absolute certainty that I had done the best I could to get pregnant. With utter earnestness, I had put forward my best effort at pregnancy, and that—my effort— was the only thing over which I had any control. Instead of hating myself for being broken or not trying hard enough, I could love myself for my valiant effort, my willingness to greet the lessons that had been served to me along the journey, and the life circumstances that had led me to this place.

Suddenly it was one hundred percent clear to me that my ability to get pregnant didn't hinge on whether or not I had a glass of wine or practiced Qigong several hours a day. In fact, I realized I may have very little, if any, control at all over pregnancy. Though the hyper-achieving, independent, lawyer part of my personality was loath to admit it, I could not *will* a pregnancy into being. If I was going to get pregnant with my own eggs, it was going to take a miracle of sorts, in which grace interceded on my behalf. My life— and my hoped-for pregnancy—was at the mercy of something bigger than I could ever comprehend. Despite all the research, experts, gadgets, medicines, and supplements at my disposal, the creation of life remained a mysterious process. I would need to ask for help and have faith.

With that, I felt called to pray. But I don't mean prayer as I had learned it through twelve years of Catholic school. After many years of spiritual practice, to me prayer didn't mean sitting down and making a request for the specific outcome I wanted. Instead it involved a practice, in which I invited the *Shen*, or light, back to the body and then I gave up control. In other words, I could not control the outcome of Project Baby, but I could create a bright and shiny home, if you will, and hope that a life might be attracted to me.

And now my desire to pray came naturally as I sought to surrender my control over how it would all turn out and trust the outcome would be perfect. My Qigong practice had often brought me to a place of experiencing an immense beauty, so magnificent it was sometimes painful. It was what I imagined the siren song to be—pure, intense, overwhelming. Trusting in this beauty, in the perfection of all outcomes, in the larger plan I could not see—I was filled with exquisite, concentrated joy and gratitude as I gazed at the majestic redwoods and fell to my knees, bent over in what I could only call prayer.

a stream of questions

"Once you get married, we'll be able to relax, knowing that you have someone other than us to take care of you." My parents had said this to me on multiple occasions. Although they had encouraged me to attend college and pursue a career of my own, they held the archaic belief that my job as a woman was to get married and settle down. Once, my father even mentioned that he and my mother had given my sister a modest sum of money when she married, as if dangling the cash in front of my face, clarifying that I would get nothing unless I married. At the time, I was struggling financially and could have used some money, but I knew better than to push the issue. These were the parents I would tell that their unmarried daughter was trying to get knocked up with a stranger's frozen sperm.

Already I had come to expect that most, if not all, of my life choices would be met with my parents' disapproval. When I had decided to go to law school, they denigrated lawyers, asking why I would want to associate with such a greedy profession. Yet when I left my law career, they begged me to reconsider. I couldn't win. Over time, I understood that what felt like disapproval to me was actually my parents' unskillful way of expressing care and concern. They couldn't help but project their money anxieties or their fears about what other people would think onto me. My lack of a steady partner and my unpredictable career path were foreign and

therefore scary to them. If I tried to explain to them that I'd cultivated a fundamental trust that I would be okay, safe, and protected
no matter what—well, that would scare them all the more.

Even with this understanding, I still found my parents' negative responses exhausting. So, though most of my friends—and even
some people I barely knew—were aware of my efforts to get pregnant, I hadn't told my parents. I worried I might absorb their stress,
which could block my ability to get pregnant. Yet if I waited until
I was pregnant to tell them, I worried that their unclaimed stress
would be bad for my baby. In short, I dreaded the conversation.

Imagining how it would unfold, I had assumed my dad, who
held traditional Catholic values about premarital sex, would be
upset about me having a baby out of wedlock. Although no sexual
exchange would happen, I feared my parents would lump all babies
born out of wedlock into the same category: bastard child. Using
a sperm donor had been difficult enough for me to wrap my brain
around. No doubt my parents would express a similar distaste for
the process. More than anything, though, I imagined they would
worry about my ability to financially support a child alone, especially given their idea that I needed a husband to take care of me.

As much as I wished I could avoid the conversation entirely,
as Christmastime rolled around, I began to feel deceptive in my
silence. When we talked on the phone and they asked what was
going on in my life, I felt increasingly uncomfortable in my omis-
sions. "Nothing new is going on," I'd lie. "Just the same old stuff."
Or I'd emphasize how my business was doing, when it was actually
occupying very little of my headspace in comparison to the struggle to get pregnant.

I did reveal Project Baby to my sister, after I returned home
from my retreat with Zhixing in England, when she had come
to Oakland for a visit. I assumed she would try to talk me out of
my decision, but when I made my announcement, she responded
enthusiastically. "Of course. I've been expecting you to tell me
something like this for years. My earliest memories are of you
wanting a baby." But then she paused and blurted out, "Do *not* tell
Mom and Dad! They will freak out and completely disapprove. If

I were you, I'd avoid the extra stress and only tell them if you get pregnant." She advised, "But when the time comes, be ready to explain each and every aspect and put their minds at ease. Be ready to explain the rigorous medical testing that each sperm donor goes through. And explain that many women purposefully get pregnant on their own these days. Call them, drop the bomb, and then tell them you are going to give them time to cool off before you talk to them about it. Then I can call them and tell them I think it's a great idea. And I can explain to them that I was expecting you to do it alone sooner, given your childhood desire for so many kids."

I was happy to have my sister's support, but the conversation reinforced my fear of telling my parents. Yet with Christmas approaching, I decided to tell them anyway, and in person. I rehearsed my speech for much of the five-hour drive to their place, east of Lake Tahoe. As soon I arrived, the words started bubbling up in my body, urgent to come out. But each time I tried to put voice to them, fear would overtake me, washing the words back, deep into my body. This cycle continued for four straight days, until my last night, when my sister had already returned to the Bay Area. As soon as I sat down for dinner with my parents, I felt the urge to tell them rise up in me again, but the fear quickly quashed the words. If this moment passed, I would likely never do it. Ultimately, I found the motivation because my mother, at age eighty, was facing some serious health conditions. She needed a hip replacement, but because of a blood clot, she couldn't have the surgery. Her mobility had decreased significantly, and as a result, her mood was suffering. Maybe the news of a potential grandchild would provide some much-needed hope and excitement? By the time dessert rolled around, I plucked up the courage. "I'm going to tell you something that might freak you out," I told my mom and dad. Then I took a big deep breath and braced myself for their reaction, "I'm trying to have a baby on my own."

Before I could say anything else, my dad jumped in with an emphatic, "Great! I think it's a wonderful idea—"

My mother interrupted, "Oh my god, how will you afford it? Where do you get the sperm, and how much does that cost? How much are the procedures?" The barrage of money-related questions was no surprise. My mother had spoken as if on cue, just as I had imagined it for months.

"Barbara," my dad cut her off, "that's insignificant! She'll figure it out. The important thing is that she wants a baby and has always wanted one." I almost fell out of my chair. Reading my mind, or my facial expression, my dad said, "It seems like you did not expect us to react this way?"

"No," I responded. "I was really scared to tell you. I thought you'd be freaked about me doing it alone and using a sperm donor."

"Well, do you get to pick the sperm donor?" my mother asked. "How do you know whether he's healthy? Do you get to choose the race?"

I answered her questions methodically, one by one. "Yes, I picked the sperm donor, and he's been rigorously tested. He's undergone way more testing than my partner would have if I were married to him."

As I answered each question, another surfaced. Trying to answer all her questions would not satiate her desire to ask more. One concern would continue to morph into the next indiscriminately. No answer would quell her fear. "You know you won't be able to travel anymore? And you can't just go to movies. You will need to find a babysitter. Have you thought this through?"

"Yes, I know I can't travel or go to movies as easily, but I've had plenty of time to play, and I'm ready for something different. I've spent months thinking about it, and the bottom line is that no matter how illogical and inconvenient it is to have a baby, I want to be a mother." I paused, taking a sip of water to buy myself some time while I thought about what I might be able to say to stave off more questions. "Mom, are you at least happy that you will have a grandchild?"

"Of course I am, but I'm just worried about how you will manage. You still haven't told me how much it all costs."

This was a trap. On the one hand, it was none of her business, and on the other hand, I knew that whatever amount of money I mentioned, she would balk. I'd stopped giving my parents any knowledge of my financial life a long time ago, because it was too stressful for them. But I felt backed into a corner, too. Not answering her question could be worse than answering it. I'd still been keeping costs relatively low by doing home IUI's for $300 per insemination with 1-2 vials of sperm costing $800 each, but I still answered, cutting the cost of procedures in half. This little white lie, I justified, would help ease her worries some. I simply couldn't face her anxiety, so it seemed easier to put her mind at ease.

Soon my dad withdrew to the living room to watch some TV, reiterating his approval, "I think it's great, Sarah."

But my mom's relentless stream of questions continued as we cleared the table and started washing dishes. "What will people think?"

"Well, it's pretty common for women to do it alone these days. There's even a term now for women who are choosing to have a child alone, called Choice Moms or Single Moms by Choice," I explained.

As I scraped food scraps into the garbage, my mom's questions ramped up to hyper-speed. I'd attempt to get an answer out, but the next question started before my sentence ended.

"Where will you have it—at home or in a hospital? How will you get health insurance for the baby—that could be too expensive? What about your roommates and living situation? Who will you live with? How will you find someone who is willing to live with a child?" And then the worst of all questions, "What if you can't get pregnant—won't you be so devastated? How will you live with the disappointment? Wouldn't it be better not to try?"

I froze in place, holding a dish in midair. "No," I responded. "I'd rather try and know that I did everything I possibly could to get pregnant. If I don't try, I'll regret that for the rest of my life." Mom's fears—they were a bottomless pit with an insatiable hunger. It didn't matter how many questions I answered or how thoroughly, the next question would always appear.

For years, I'd been working with Chris to let go of my desire for my parents' approval, which I knew I would never get. Along the way, I learned that I could control only my experience, which meant, of course, I had to get comfortable letting my mother have *her* experience. Anxiety was an inevitable part of my mom's experience. I did not want to be callous about the stress my mother was under, but I could not manage it for her. Honestly, if she weren't stressing about my desire to have a baby alone, she'd find something else about my life to cause her anxiety. It's just how my mom was wired. This conversation, while challenging, offered an opportunity to practice remaining calm and committed to my truth in the face of someone else's anxiety. Energetically, I stayed centered in my own being, rather than merging with my mother and trying to lessen her anxiety for her. I saw this as a vital skill for motherhood, so I welcomed the opportunity to practice.

The next morning, I set off for the Bay Area. As I drove away, I felt tremendous relief. I couldn't believe that my mom and dad were on board, and, amidst the concerns, they were genuinely happy for me. It was a rare experience for me. I was not going to have to fight against their disapproval after all. That said, I knew I would not be calling up my mother to share my journey with her. I knew the ups and downs, which were almost too much for me to handle at times, would certainly be too much for her. Instead I'd titrate information to her, as needed. This was nothing new. Since I was a young girl, my mother's inability to manage her own feelings, let alone mine, had forced me to become emotionally independent, and nothing had changed on this front. In fact, this self-reliance empowered me to know that I could handle anything life brought my way, even a baby, even on my own.

the last ditch effort— medical intervention

By mid-January, I was still attempting to approach Project Baby with my internal compass—not some set of externally prescribed rules—as my guide. In my attempt to "try with less fervor," I learned there was a fine line between "trying without trying" and "giving up." One morning, I sat on the edge of my bed, unable to meet my day. My body felt totally wrecked, and my psyche was a deflated balloon lying in the corner, days after the party, wilted and gathering dust. *I should just give up. Trying to be a mother is just too hard. I'm done.* I couldn't imagine mustering up the hope and faith necessary to enter yet another IUI cycle, only to be crushed by a negative result a few weeks later. I allowed myself to be swept away by visions of myself lying on the beach, soaking up sun, sipping margaritas, and going out salsa dancing in the warm, perfect nights. I could imagine myself having fun again, living a carefree, unencumbered life. Maybe my mother was right—it was too devastating to try only to fail.

But as soon as I let that pendulum swing all the way to the "no baby" side, it swung back to reality: I wanted a baby. If this was what it required to become a mother, I needed to dust myself off and try again. I needed to reach into the depths of my being to find the courage and energy to continue. If I didn't, I'd regret it for the rest of my life. The limbo—not knowing *if* it would happen, not knowing *when* it would happen, not knowing what more I would need to go through to *make* it happen—this was taking its toll on me. It was time to figure out which steps I still needed to take before I could say I'd done my best to try to get pregnant with my own eggs, before I moved on to some other option, like egg donation. I thought back over all of my attempts to time inseminations properly. I'd done my best to enhance and track my fertility, and I'd done my best to make sure I was actually ovulating, even though it was unclear whether or not I was. What was next? If I consulted a Reproductive Endocrinologist (RE), I could do a medicated IUI cycle. The RE would prescribe Clomid, or some other drug, to hyperstimulate my ovaries and precisely time ovulation. With the combination of an ultrasound—to see the follicle ripening—and a trigger shot—to force ovulation when the follicle was mature—an RE might be able to increase my odds of getting pregnant using my own eggs.

In the past, I'd been loath to try any Western drugs. I'd heard many horror stories about Clomid, which is often the first fertility drug administered. I thought of it as the gateway fertility drug, since it was practically given out like candy to any woman who encountered any trouble getting pregnant. As I understood it, Clomid was notorious for causing ovarian cysts, weight gain, and other mysterious side effects, so I had bristled at the thought of using it when I had just begun my journey. But now, when I tried to envision my ovaries, I saw rusty pieces of broken-down machinery. The risk of developing cysts on those heaps of junk seemed inconsequential.

I thought back to the appointment I'd had with an RE five months earlier. I'd sat in her office, feeling the empty chair next to me that normally would have been occupied by a partner, listening to her gloomy prognosis. According to my blood tests, all three measures of fertility looked abysmal. My FSH, AMH, and resting follicle count were all consistent with menopause. "With your numbers," she had explained, "I can't recommend any treatment. If you had one bad number, we might try some treatments. But all of your numbers are quite bad. Your only real chance is to go for an egg donor." At the time, I hadn't understood whether the reproductive endocrinologist refused to give me Clomid or other treatments because of the risk that any baby conceived with such bad numbers would be disabled, or whether it was just because she figured it would be a waste of time and money. Or was it a more sinister motivation to refuse to treat women who were unlikely to be successful to keep their success statistics high? Regardless, by mid-January I decided it was time to pull out all the stops. I called the RE assigned to me at the fertility clinic to clarify her rationale and to find out what treatment options might be available.

When I got her on the phone, she explained, "You can try a medicated cycle with Clomid, but it is very unlikely that it will work, given your numbers. I support you to do whatever you need to do to have closure and move on to an egg donor. I know this is different for every woman, and you should do what you feel is necessary."

I appreciated her bluntness. I wasn't turned off by the idea that Clomid would be a long shot. My whole journey had been a long shot. Though I'd wrestled mightily along the way, the journey itself had its benefits: I was grateful for the life lessons I had encountered. In the end, I needed to know I had at least tried Clomid before I started looking at egg donation. I simply wasn't ready to go there yet. So I asked for the protocol. On day three of my cycle I would start taking Clomid for three to five days, which would hopefully force my ovaries to ripen as many eggs as possible. The doctor's technician would do an ultrasound on day fourteen to monitor the progress of the follicles. Once the eggs reached a certain maturity, measured by their size, the doctor would administer an HCG injection to trigger ovulation so that the IUI could be precisely timed just before ovulation. Immediately following, I would start a high dose of progesterone to mimic the hormones that my body should naturally be creating if it were performing properly.

With that, I bought my ticket to the Clomid train. To move forward, the RE's patient coordinator sent me an email with fourteen pages of consents and waivers that needed to be notarized. I fasted the next morning for a complete panel of blood tests, including an HIV test, syphilis, Hep B, cholesterol panel, and full metabolic panel. The financial assistant also contacted me with an agreement and breakdown of fees which amounted to roughly $3000, asking for partial payment of the treatment up front. I checked all these boxes on the to-do list right away. I was ready. Except I had no idea what part of my cycle I was in. I'd continued to have weird, mid-cycle bleeding and no periods. Thanks to my rebellion, I was no longer taking my temperature or monitoring the other signs I'd so diligently tracked in the past. I had no clue when I was going to ovulate next. Luckily, my period answered that question by showing up a few days later, and I began the highest possible dosage of Clomid for five days.

I was completely wired during those days. I couldn't sleep and felt like my heart was beating out of my chest. But, in the big scheme of things, I didn't care. As I lay awake at night, I reviewed the doctor's instructions. I was supposed to start doing OPKs on day eleven by 8:30 A.M. If the kit detected an LH surge, I was supposed to call the office immediately and make an appointment for an ultrasound that day. If I did not get a positive OPK by day fourteen, I was supposed to call and schedule an ultrasound for day fifteen. I could see so many problems with this plan. First, I'd never had a clearly positive OPK. By now, I had tried six or seven brands, all of which returned inconsistent results. To say I was uncomfortable relying on OPKs would be an understatement. I'd explained to the nurse assigned to assist me through the process that I was very good at tracking my cervix and noticing when it was soft, that'd I do the OPKs but I wanted to rely on my cervix texture instead, she dismissed me, instructing me to rely on the "objective" test. How could she discount my own sense of my body in favor of a test that had proven unreliable for me? No wonder women were so divorced from their bodies in the age of modern medicine.

And that wasn't the only problem. Historically, I had ovulated on day eleven or twelve. So even if Clomid extended my cycle, as it was prone to do, waiting until day fifteen for the first ultrasound seemed ludicrous. I sent my nurse coordinator several messages to this effect, and she promised to ask the doctor, but by day twelve, I learned that she had failed to ask. Later that day, the nurse coordinator told me to schedule my ultrasound for day twelve. However, the office only scheduled ultrasounds in the early morning, so I'd missed the window for that day. I immediately scheduled for early morning day thirteen. I knew my cervix was still quite firm on day twelve, so I assumed I'd be okay. When I arrived to the office expectant and eager, my hope was dampened by the attitude of nurses and technicians. As I climbed onto the examining table, the tech asked, "You're here for your LH surge sono? You had a positive OPK?" I had to bite my tongue as I responded, "No, I haven't had a positive OPK yet." I began filling her in on the details of my short cycles, cervical changes, and current ovulation pain. "I am here to make sure I am not going to miss ovulation and to check the follicles."

"What side did you feel ovulation pain on?" she asked, seeming to ignore all of the self-reported information about my tracking. She was only interested in OPKs.

"On the right," I responded. I felt like I was being tested, and she wasn't listening to me.

I spread my legs and she inserted the phallic probe to look at my ovaries. After a few moments she reported, "You have a follicle at 20 mm on the right and nothing on the left. I guess you were correct that the ovulation pains were on the right. I am always surprised when women know their bodies well enough to feel on which side they are ovulating." She gave me a smirk and nervous laugh.

I gritted my teeth and tried not to lose my temper. I was so sick of telling everyone at this office that I *knew* my body, only to be dismissed.

Then she continued, "Your lining is thin. Only 5 mm. Ideally we like it to be about 7-8 mm minimum but 10 or more is ideal. I'm going to see if I can reach the doctor to ask whether there is something we can do to help your lining. Get dressed and wait here. I'll be back in a minute, after I call your doctor."

I got dressed and patiently waited. Thirty minutes later, the nurse returned to tell me that she couldn't find the doctor. "Someone will call you within the hour," she assured me. Before she could rush back out the door, I stopped her to ask when she anticipated the insemination might take place, so I could make plans for my tank. "I have a tank with my sperm samples inside in my car. I was wondering if you might be able to refill it with dry ice if necessary?"

"Oh, that's so cute. Is it like a security blanket?" she responded. "You like to have it close by at all times?"

I wanted to slap her, but instead I calmly explained, "I have been working with a midwife who will come to my house any time day or night to get the timing just right. I don't want to be beholden to the hours your offices are available to do an IUI, so I am storing the tank with me instead of here at your offices." I had lost my motivation to get the tank topped off with dry ice. Instead, I walked out, not hiding my displeasure.

I went home frustrated by my experience, but excited that I had a good follicle. I was anxious for the doctor to call in an estrogen prescription, so that I could start thickening my lining. I was acutely aware that I didn't have much time, since my follicle was already at 20 mm. As soon as I got home, I emailed my nurse coordinator to make sure she knew the doctor was supposed to call me. But after several hours, I still hadn't heard from the nurse or the doctor. All day I stuck close to my phone and postponed errands, so I could be able to fill a prescription at a moment's notice. An ominous feeling started to creep over me, though, as the hour grew later and the doctor still hadn't called me back. Around two I called the nurse coordinator again. "The doctor should call you in less than an hour," she responded. By four o'clock the doctor still hadn't called, and I was pissed. If I was going to be able to do something to thicken my lining, it needed to happen as quickly as possible. By four, I could have been taking estrogen for more than eight hours. By five o'clock, I was livid. But under the rumblings of my angry mind, my heart and gut knew something was up—this was happening for a reason. Finally, around five-thirty the phone rang. I recognized the area code and answered quickly. I knew from the tone of her voice as she said hello that the doctor did not have good news.

"I'm sorry, Sarah, but we have to call off this cycle. Your lining is just too thin for how advanced your follicle is." There it was, the bad news. "One of the known side effects of Clomid is that it thins the uterine lining. So, we can try a different drug next cycle."

I wanted to jump through the phone to strangle her. We had lost an entire valuable day. If I'd been able to start the estrogen that morning, I might have had a chance. What's more, the doctor had never mentioned that Clomid could thin the uterine lining, and I was irritated that this crucial information had been omitted. I knew my body well enough that I could have warned her that my lining was likely to be thin. At my first appointment, she had even mentioned that my lining was paper thin, but she never bothered to ask me any questions that might have revealed that Clomid was not the best choice for me. Why hadn't she given me the alternate drug to begin with, or started monitoring my lining earlier? Once again, I felt like I was bumping up against an industry that assumed no one knew any details about their own bodies. They simply followed a generic protocol, even when the patient knew her own body. Clearly, I was part of a factory.

Instead of voicing my displeasure, though, I managed to remain calm and polite. I hung up the phone and burst into tears. A mix of despair and frustration swirled through me. I flopped onto my bed as the tears flowed. My dogs, sensing I was upset, jumped on the bed and nuzzled in beside me as I wept.

the miracle
(or so i thought)

A few hours later, I wiped away my tears and rolled out of bed. Unbelievably, I had a date that night. I still felt tender, but I knew the distraction would pull me out of the puddle of tears and agony. I poured a cocktail and jumped in the shower to primp.

In early December, I had started dating Jay, a friend from the salsa world. We had flirted for years, but he took it up a notch one night when he sent me a playful text message. I responded in kind, and we started hanging out that week. In the heart of my rebellion, the timing seemed perfect. At first, we saw each other about once a week, a combination of late-night visits and proper dates. Within a month, it became twice a week. I went into this situation thinking it was just a casual last hurrah before getting pregnant and being tied down by a baby. But now that Jay and I were spending more time together, I was starting to fantasize about him sticking around while I made a baby. Or better yet, I daydreamed about him giving me his sperm. I knew I was getting ahead of myself, but I had been through a difficult year alone, and it was easy to get carried away and romanticize a perfect partnership resulting in a love child.

However, I had not told Jay about my pregnancy attempts, and I was torturing myself with the question of when and what to tell him. Withholding this information about the biggest decision of my life, while trying to cultivate intimacy with Jay, felt awkward at best. I consulted the Choice Moms message boards seeking guidance and found no one knew the answer to this ubiquitous question, though all agreed: it felt weird.

I recalled the conversation I'd had with Rodrigo, whom I'd been casually dating even after I had started trying to conceive. When I told him I wanted to have a baby on my own, he thought it was utterly cool. Having been raised in Mexico City, entrenched in the Catholic Church and conservative views about the family structure, he was fascinated by alternative approaches to life. As a forty-year old man, he'd been pressured by women he was dating to have another family. In contrast, if I wanted a baby on my own and wasn't asking him for anything in return, he was not only supportive but intrigued. "I love babies," he'd remarked gleefully. "After you have a baby, I'll visit. I can get my baby fix. After you put the baby to bed, we can have our fun together." To him it seemed modern and cool, and it didn't sound too bad in my book either.

But I wasn't sure Jay was going to have the same laissez-faire reaction. I feared that telling him I was trying to get pregnant would transform our budding relationship in his eyes, from a flirtatious, salsa-dancing partnership turned love affair, to that of a lion tamer coaxing her king of the jungle into a cage. Though I had no intention of caging Jay into the responsibilities of parenthood, if Jay wasn't ready to be around a baby, I was afraid he might push me away. I needed some laughter and distraction from the difficult year I'd had. It was so much easier to blow off my disappointment when I had a lovely person to look forward to seeing. Not to mention I wanted to have fun before my body would change forever (and not, as I had been warned, for the better) and I had a screaming baby in the next room. So I continued to vacillate back and forth, Project Baby looming like a silent partner in the room.

"Sarah, we have some surprising news," the doctor said, joy reverberating in his voice. "You're pregnant. That's right, you're pregnant!" I almost fell over. My whole body began to shake as I held my phone. I had just completed the first day of a weekend Qigong workshop. Chris, Genevieve, and Vicki were deciding where to go to lunch, while I checked my voicemail. I was walking toward them as the doctor's words shimmered through my body. They could tell something was up. "What's wrong? Are you okay?" Genevieve asked.

As I slid my phone into my pocket, I blurted out the most improbable news, "I'm pregnant." I watched their jaws drop open as I began to shake and cry, gasping for air as they congratulated me. The ultimate miracle had happened. I had attained the one-percent chance at pregnancy.

But how in the world could I be pregnant? I hadn't had a period since before taking the Clomid. When I had called the fertility clinic to ask what to do, they recommended a blood test to better predict when and whether to start a new round of drugs. "But, you will also have to do a pregnancy test. It's just protocol," the nurse coordinator had explained. My last insemination with donor sperm had been over three months ago. In the meantime, I'd been sleeping with Jay, but we had been careful. Now the doctor's voicemail was telling me I was pregnant? It could only mean one thing: I was pregnant with Jay's baby. I must have conceived on February 26, my birthday, roughly two weeks prior. Jay and I hadn't seen each other since then. I thought back to our last conversation in which he had explained his distance, "I'm too overwhelmed to be physically and emotionally involved right now." Well, if he thought the rest of his life was overwhelming, I was about to drop the ultimate bomb on him. Even knowing how much this would stress him out, I could not curtail my elation.

Standing on a street corner was no way to celebrate, so we decided to go to lunch. I was so excited and shocked that Genevieve had to drive my car. The whole way across city traffic on that glorious sunny day, we marveled at the news. "I did it," I kept saying. My hard work and practice had finally paid off. I got my miracle.

As soon as I calmed down a bit, I noticed another voicemail on my phone—a nurse from the RE's office. At the sound of her voice, I bristled. My heart sank, my guts did a flip. Yet the message simply explained that I needed to repeat the blood tests and start taking progesterone to support the pregnancy. *Why do they want me to repeat the blood test?* I questioned, but then I remembered it was standard procedure to take two blood tests, forty-eight hours apart, to make sure the pregnancy was proceeding normally. Relief washed over me, but still, something in the nurse's tone made me nervous. Because it was a Saturday, the office was already closed, so I couldn't call back to get the instructions and progesterone prescription. Instead, I carried on with my celebrations.

Later that day, on my drive home, I called my friend Andrea, an OB/GYN from Chile, who was living in Berkeley, completing a master's in Public Health. When I told her the news, I could hear her voice quaver, fighting back tears as she cooed her congratulations in Spanish. Unable to contain my good news, when I arrived home, I called Annette. We spent over an hour on the phone, figuring out the due date and the astrological sign of the coming baby. I confessed that I wanted to jump up immediately and go to the consignment baby store to pick out a stroller. Annette, who had two grown boys and a grandson, fantasized about it being a girl. When I explained that it had to be Jay's, we marveled over how cute the baby would be. All the while, I knew it was risky to tell other people so early. But since I had no significant other and a distant relationship with my family, connecting with my friends, whom I kept up to date about every turn of events, was my way of being seen in the world, of staying in touch with witnesses and support.

After a few more phone calls, I laid down in my zero-gravity chair in the garden. It was unseasonably warm, at least 70 degrees in the middle of March. As the sun warmed my skin, I drifted in and out as an amazing softness came over me. I was overcome by intense love for myself. I was not a failure as a woman. I was a fully functioning woman. I would be a mother! I had proved my practice, dedication, and faith. I was brimming over with pride, love, and kindness. When I thought about the baby growing inside me, I was filled with an intense motivation to shower myself with tenderness. I firmly believed that because my thoughts and emotions affected my biochemistry, they would affect the baby growing inside me. Abiding in love and kindness as much as possible would be a gift to my baby. I spoke to the baby. "You are so loved and perfect. A true miracle. The answer to my prayers. I will love you with all my heart."

I spent the rest of my day floating in ecstasy. That night, I tossed and turned with excitement. But I was also starting to worry about telling Jay. Throughout each of my conversations with my friends, the same question had surfaced, "When are you going to tell Jay?" I would wait to make sure the pregnancy was progressing before I told him. I did not want to worry him unnecessarily.

I knew the news would not be well received. My main concern was the seeming contradiction in my story—that although I had been trying to get pregnant on my own for months, getting pregnant with his baby truly was an accident. We'd been using condoms and I hadn't ovulated in god knows how long. I needed to convey the mistake and the miracle in equal measure. How could I communicate both the strength of my conviction to be pregnant and the truth that I had not tried to trap him? Would I be able to explain that I had been willing to do it alone using a sperm donor, so he did not feel pressure to be involved? I could not change the fact that he was the father of my child, but I could give him complete choice and freedom about whether he wanted to be involved. Of course, I would be thrilled if he did want to be involved, but I needed him to understand that I would not be upset if he decided not to be.

After a few hours of tossing and turning, I gave up on sleep and went online to read about pregnancy. I learned what I could not eat and how much weight I should gain, and I started searching for names. I registered for updates about my baby's growth and development on not one but three online sites. I even started reading about the personality of Scorpios, the astrological sign for the baby's due date.

On Sunday morning, I called the nurse to get details about starting progesterone, and I took the opportunity to get more information. She went over the labs with me and reported that my

HCG was 461. HCG is a chemical produced by your body as soon as a fertilized egg implants into the uterine wall, so its presence is used to detect pregnancy. It doubles every two days for the first few weeks. "Based on your HCG levels, I'd guess that you conceived about two and a half weeks ago." I gulped—that was exactly my birthday. "We want you to repeat the HCG on Monday. It's standard procedure," she explained. I breathed a sigh of relief. She seemed calm and unconcerned.

I floated through the rest of my day at Qigong class, beaming and elated.

On Monday morning, I awoke early to get the blood test at the first possible opportunity. It was another gloriously sunny day, so after the blood test, I grabbed the dogs and headed up into the hills. On my drive back home, I called another close friend to tell her the news. I was contemplating who else to call, but decided I should hold off until I got the blood tests back. I didn't want to jinx myself by entertaining any doubt about losing the baby, but I also knew it was unusual to share news of pregnancy so early. Soon after returning from my walk, I sat down in my kitchen to eat a burrito. The phone rang, and I recognized the doctor's office area code, so I picked up as fast as I could. The minute I heard the doctor's voice, I knew. I expected she would say I had lost the baby. But the news was even more disturbing. "I'm sorry, Sarah," she said, "you are not pregnant and were actually never pregnant. The lab switched your results with someone else's."

I couldn't speak, so she kept talking. "We reran your blood samples from Friday and today," she explained. "Your levels of progesterone and estrogen are too low for pregnancy and you have no HCG in your blood at all."

I had a million questions, but I couldn't think clearly enough to decipher them. I hurried to get off the phone. The ground pulled away from me. I couldn't breathe. Before the full force of the shock could hit me, I quickly shot off a text message, cutting and pasting the same message to save time, telling my friends it was all a mistake. For some reason, it felt urgent for them all to know the truth immediately. I did not want anyone to think I was pregnant for any longer than necessary.

I scarfed down my burrito, keeping the tears at bay while I distractedly swallowed. It gave me something to do while I processed the information. Then I hurried up to my room, turned off my ringer, and fell into bed. The tears started to flow. I sobbed until I exhausted myself into sleep. From time to time, I awoke and cried again until I fell asleep. I slept and cried for the next three hours. I wanted to hide and never see the world again. I wanted to know who was playing this cruel joke on me. Of course it would be devastating to be pregnant and lose the baby. But given my crazy odds of getting pregnant, it seemed worse to have the news that I was never pregnant. There was no miracle, and there probably wouldn't be one. I vowed to give up, feeling certain that I couldn't muster the strength to carry on. Was this slap in the face sent to help me realize I wasn't meant to be a mother?

I awoke a few hours later. Many friends had texted and called repeatedly. I forced myself to respond to a few text messages, and I spoke to one or two friends. I didn't know what to do next. Being idle felt dangerous. I dragged myself into my garden to bury myself in a task.

About a year prior, I'd fired my gardener and bought a manual push mower. It wasn't very effective, and over time my lawn had become a pocked landscape of bald dirt and clumps of long grass. In the past month, that grass had grown eight inches. The push mower just ran over the top of it, flattening down the tufts, refusing to cut it. This was the perfect task. I turned my iPhone on for some music, and I knelt in the garden with my largest kitchen knife, cutting each clump of grass by hand. When I finished this, I would add compost to the holes, sprinkling a little seed on top, and fitting a custom-cut piece of sod over each open space. I spent hours engrossed in my project. I dreaded ever having to speak to anyone ever again. The only silver lining was I didn't have to drag Jay through the whole experience. Yet this too added to my sense of loss. Having believed the baby was Jay's—someone I knew instead of an anonymous sperm donor—had been such a boost for me. Losing that unexpected boost made it feel so much harder to go on alone.

After I don't know how long, my roommate came home and found me in the yard. I can't imagine how I looked, hunched with my knife, cutting each blade of grass individually. It was getting late, and I was cold and wet, my back aching from leaning over.

"How can I help you?" she asked.

"I need someone to feed me," I said. "I can't function on that level right now. And please tell anyone you might have told what happened that I do not under any circumstances want to discuss it with them."

Now I understood why people were cautious about spreading pregnancy news. Because when the devastation hits, it's hard to face people, even people you love. It's impossible to control how people respond. In my case, some people called and texted right away. Others were mysteriously silent, waiting a few days to say anything or not responding at all. Either way, the responses felt inadequate, unfair, and insensitive, because really, what can anyone say to appease this kind of shock and grief? I knew that I would tell all the important people in my life one day, but this need to report anything right away felt grossly uncomfortable. After my roommate made me some soup, and I drowned my sorrows in a few Manhattans, I fell asleep wishing I could wake up in three months, after all this had blown over.

nothing except love
makes sense

*M*y alarm rang at 6:30 A.M., a sound met by a lump in my throat and an ache in my heart. Two days after the floor dropped out underneath my supposed pregnancy, I was heading to a Qigong retreat.

Entering the practice room, I carried my head down, surrounding myself with an energetic bubble to keep people away. Though I was yearning for some recognition of my pain, I dreaded seeing friends who knew what had happened. I wanted sympathy, but I felt so raw I didn't want to talk.

When class started, Chris instructed us to get blankets for a Feldenkrais Awareness Through Movement (ATM) lesson. We laid on our backs with our knees bent and our feet standing flat on the ground, shoulder width apart. Chris gave the first instruction, "Slowly tilt your legs to the right. Notice how your pelvis moves and notice how the ribs move. What inhibits this movement?"

A new student raised her hand and told Chris, "I can't lay on my back because I'm too far along in my pregnancy."

A dagger plunged into my heart. Of course, this would be the first retreat a pregnant woman attended. And of course her blanket would be a few feet away from mine. Chris took a break from the lesson to advise her. I tried hard not to listen. Just hearing any reference to her pregnancy felt physically painful. I spent the remainder of the session feeling irritated and angry at everyone and everything.

After lunch, we debriefed our first session. As a student shared her joy over a personal realization, I held my tongue and gripped my chair, quelling an impulse to slap that joy off her face. I knew my anger and irritation were misplaced. Of course I was angry not at my fellow students but at the doctors and the lab. They had seriously screwed up, and I was furious. Someone needed to explain what had gone wrong. Who was at fault: the clinic or the lab? Didn't the doctors suspect that the first results were incorrect, since the numbers were so inconsistent? Some of the blood work indicated pregnancy, while other numbers would have been impossible if I had been pregnant. My mind sped through these questions like a hamster on a wheel, stirring up rage. *The responsible party should pay for this mistake*, I thought. *Otherwise, it's simply not fair.*

I sought out Chris for counsel. "How do I reconcile this anger? I know that I'm justified being mad at the doctors, but I can also see that doesn't help me. How do I deal with it?"

Chris pointed to my words *justified* and *fair.* "As long as you hold on to this notion, you'll be miserable. Life isn't fair, so seeking justice is a dead-end street. Can you let go of the injustice and accept it was a mistake in order to move on? Instead seek the lesson being taught?"

This counsel—to release attachment to justice or fairness— was not new to me. When I first met Chris, I was freshly out of practicing law. I could win any argument and reason my way out of anything, claiming my perspective was just and correct. "I am not determined to be right out of sheer stubbornness, but justice demands this outcome," I would argue. "It's simply a matter of principle."

Chris would laugh and say to me, "Do you want to be right or do you want to be happy?"

"Why can't I be right and happy?" I would respond. "They aren't mutually exclusive." It took me years to understand what he meant.

Since then I had learned that clinging to the rightness of my position left me feeling justified, but at too great a cost. This strange concept, justice, applied only to the material world. On an esoteric level or matters of the heart, who can say what is "right"? In the big scheme of things, we cannot judge if an experience is "right" or "wrong." We only know it happened.

Here I was again, facing that old conundrum. I could continue to stay angry at the doctors. I could figure out who was responsible—the clinic or the lab? I could track down the guilty parties and let them know how they hurt me. I knew better than to think a lawsuit would be a good idea or even possible, but I could pursue "justice" through social media and online reviews. Or I could see that the doctors, like everyone else in the universe, were doing the best they could. I could even try to love them instead of resenting them. I knew this to be true intellectually, but in practice this remained a lofty concept that I couldn't yet adopt. I was still angry, and I needed to point a finger at someone.

Later that day, we sat in a circle discussing our experience with practice. Angela raised her hand, "I realized in that meditation, how much I love my dantien." We all started laughing at the ridiculousness of this statement. But in that moment, the love she felt was palpable and contagious. A phrase popped into in my head, *Nothing except love makes sense. Nothing except love makes sense. Nothing except love makes sense.* I couldn't turn it off. Right or wrong no longer mattered; the only thing that made sense was love.

As the mantra played on, I was overcome by love for the doctors. I had been lucky enough to realize a few months ago that *I* was doing my best, but now it was my chance to see that everyone around me—they too were doing their best. They wanted nothing more than for me to be pregnant. As I opened love to them, I opened to loving myself. The tenderness and self-love that flooded me when I thought I was pregnant returned in full force. This was the way. This was why it felt like someone had played what seemed an incredibly mean trick, so I could learn the greatest lesson of this lifetime: to be kind to myself. Since the last retreat, I had practice replacing self-loathing with kindness. I'd already softened my stance by recognizing that I had done my best, but while I thought I was pregnant I'd experienced a deeper, truer, more complete self-love. I'd lavished in its softness and learned it contours. Now it was bookmarked in my psyche and my body. Now I knew not only how to find it, but how to abide in it.

part 3: arriving

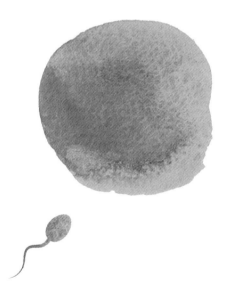

clarity

The missed miracle marked a shift for me: I began to let go of the hope that my own eggs might be viable. When I got home from the retreat, I started researching egg donation. I wanted time to digest the information and mull over my options, while watching where I had energy to move forward and noting where I felt blocked. Instead of choosing one path toward pregnancy and walking it, though, I took both routes simultaneously, pouring my mental energy into preparing for my next IUI cycle, while exploring egg donation options. Living of two minds exhausted me, but I was forty-two. It had been two exhausting years since I first opened the question of single motherhood, and I had no time to lose. If I didn't conceive during my upcoming medicated IUI with an alternative drug to Clomid called Letrozole, I wanted to be ready to launch Plan C: Egg Donor. (I'd already used Plan B when I decided to have a baby without a partner).

I had thought preparing to use a sperm donor felt strange, but that was nothing compared to the journey toward egg donation. I knew I was having an emotional reaction to the idea of using an egg donor, but I had never tried to untangle it and understand its foundations. I knew from my coach training that asking hard questions, and continuing to follow the answers with more questions, could help me tease apart any undifferentiated thoughts and emotions. So I began asking. At Chris's suggestion, I started by asking myself why I so wanted a genetic connection to a child. What did it mean for my child to share my genes or not? Was this desire rooted in a notion of natural selection—I wanted to pass on *my* genes? Was my desire hardwired in me as biological self-preservation? No, the need to pass on any genetic advantages in my family line did not feel relevant in modern day society. Sure, I had fears about the unknown aspects of a donor's genetics, but that was a far cry from needing to pass on my own genes for the preservation of the species.

Did I want to use my own eggs simply because I had always assumed I would have a genetic link to my child, from the first moment I understood how babies were made? For most people, the desire for a genetic connection is deeply rooted in assumptions about family—blood is thicker than water and all that. But my emotional ties to the people I called family were certainly not dependent on a genetic connection. Indeed, I was closer to my chosen family and friends, with whom I shared no genetic connection, than to anyone in my biological family.

Even still, the magic of gazing at my future baby, seeing myself in him or her—this was something I had dreamed of as a child. When I took the time to examine it closely though, I could see this was an egoist emotional desire. On the flip side, what would it mean not to be able to see myself in my child? Did it mean I wanted to forgo motherhood? Definitely not.

Ultimately I came to see my knee-jerk reaction against using an egg donor as an undifferentiated emotional attachment. My desire for a genetically related child was nothing more than an attachment to the way I thought things should be.

Even still, I was apprehensive about using both a sperm and an egg donor. I assumed that the vast majority of women who contemplated using an egg donor were in a partnership, thus the child maintained a genetic link to one person in the equation. In my case, there would be no genetic link, making it more like adoption. So why wasn't I contemplating adoption?

I was trying to honor my gut impulses when they arose, and—short answer—I couldn't muster the energy to research it after hearing that it was extremely difficult, though not impossible, for a single woman to adopt. It also didn't help that I'd heard a few horror stories from friends and acquaintances in the last few years. I'd had a friend who had adopted the previous year and seen how emotionally difficult the uncertainty of process had been for her. Once, she got a call in the night that they had a baby for her. She and her husband jumped on a plane, only to arrive to a birth mother who wanted to keep her baby. Though I never did any extensive research, the cost sounded prohibitively expensive. Other's had presented the adoption question as well.

When I told a former housemate I might need to use both an egg and sperm donor, she'd asked, "Why don't you just adopt?" The judgment implicit in her question shocked me, and I fumbled for an answer. Before I could open my mouth, she said, "I'm sorry. I just believe very strongly in adoption, so your choice makes no sense to me. It's essentially like adopting anyways, since the baby will be completely unrelated to you."

I took a deep breath, settling myself. How could I blame her for posing the same question I'd been asking myself? If we were both having this reaction, how many others would as well? Did I want to face this question, on a broad scale, for the entirety of my child's life?

"Is it just that you really want to experience pregnancy?" she pressed.

"I do. I really want to be pregnant and to breastfeed," I confirmed.

I knew this with absolute certainty, not so much because I wanted to gain forty pounds or suffer back aches and swollen feet, or endure the overwhelming need to pee every five minutes, but because I believed that carrying a baby in my body for nine-and-a-half months would link us in profound ways, physically, emotionally, and perhaps even genetically. After all, he'd be bathing in my juices, experiencing my emotions, tasting my food, and smelling my odors. Just like all the nutrients I would be eating, my biochemistry would pass through the placenta to the baby. Every time I danced, sang, or practiced Qigong, he would experience my rhythm, sounds, and joy.

Turns out this gut instinct had a scientific basis. A burgeoning field called fetal origins, or maternal effects research, examines the effects of stress, diet, pharmaceuticals, chemicals, and pollutants on the health of a fetus while it's developing in the womb, at birth, and throughout life. In her book, *Origins: How the Nine Months Before Birth Shape the Rest of Our Lives*, Annie Murphy Paul writes, "The pregnant woman is neither a passive incubator nor a source of always imminent harm to her fetus, but a powerful and often positive influence on her child even before it's born." Fetal origins research has revealed that a pregnant woman's daily life—the air she breathes, the food and drink she consumes, the emotions she feels, the stress she endures, and the chemicals she is exposed to—are shared with the fetus and taken by the fetus as "biological postcards from the outside world." In short, the conditions in utero play a major role in creating a foundation for health, intelligence, and temperament.

Shortly after I started seriously considering egg donors, I was sitting at a bar with my friend Jose, a neuroscientist visiting from Chile. I shared my journey with Jose—my difficulty getting pregnant, as well as my concerns about using an egg donor.

Jose stopped me mid-sentence, full of excitement, "Don't worry about using an egg donor at all. Carrying him in your body plays an enormous role in which genes your baby expresses. It's epigenetics!" This friend I lovingly call the Mad Scientist became so excited his voice drowned out a group of loud girls next to us. "It's a relatively new field in the study of human inheritance," Jose continued. "Epigenetics literally means 'above or on top of the genome.'" According to Jose, scientists have discovered that tags of information, usually methyl groups, form on DNA, altering the behavior of a gene, causing it to express or not to express. Just as I had suspected, dietary and environmental factors, such as stress and chemical exposure, and the uterine environment cause these tags to form. Scientists now believe the DNA sequence itself is much less important than once thought. The fate of cells in the embryo depends not only on the genome (DNA) but also on the environment that each of the developing cells sense during prenatal development and throughout life. The environment, however, both before and after birth, plays a pivotal role in genetic expression. Jose concluded his mini-lecture, "My prediction is that within the next ten to twenty years, we will discover that our genetic code only accounts for a small percentage of what actually gets inherited and what makes us who we are."

That night, I left the bar educated and uplifted, hopeful and determined to learn as much as I could about epigenetics. As soon as I got home, I turned to Google to read articles and even purchased several books on the subject. I quickly learned that in the last decade, our concept of DNA has vastly expanded. DNA is no longer viewed as a template that produces identical copies of the same thing. The genes still need instructions for what to do and where to do it. One of the most conclusive studies illustrating epigenetic changes due to uterine conditions is the agouti mouse study, which was first published in *Molecular and Cellular Biology* in 2003. The mice were bred to be genetically identical to each other with the agouti gene coding for brown fur. Those mice that were exposed to certain chemicals such as bisphenol-A (or BPA, which occurs in some types of household plastic) and poor diets in utero were born not with the brown fur coded in their genes, but with *yellow* fur. They were also prone to diabetes, obesity, and cancer.

This blew my mind! What might this mean for my future child? This new information had huge implications for any woman using an egg donor. If I chose egg donation, I would not be the genetic mother, but as the biological mother, I would help shape my baby's physical and mental development. For a pregnant woman, this seems an enormous responsibility to bear, and the lawyer in me recognized that this argument about gestational influence had its dangers. But as a recipient of another woman's egg, I felt reassured beyond measure knowing that I could be a big part of the equation. I was not solely at the mercy of my donors' DNA. She would provide the blueprint, but I would provide the building materials and do the construction. Every cell of the baby's body would be built out of my proteins, sugars, calcium, and fluids.

In the end, I knew I could get comfortable giving up my DNA. It wasn't what I wanted to do, but the prospect no longer felt devastating.

When I got my next period, I had to charge up enough stamina for what I had promised myself would be my last IUI. Though I felt reassured by my back-up plan, I was dreading this cycle. This time I would take Letrozole to stimulate my ovaries, which does not thin the uterine lining as Clomid was prone to do. The doctor and I also planned to check my lining and follicles on day ten, so we'd have more time to thicken my lining if necessary. This tricky dance would require perfect timing—if I started estrogen too soon it could inhibit follicle growth, but if I started too late my lining wouldn't thicken enough before ovulation.

By the time day ten rolled around, I was anxious as a mama cat at a dog show, ready to pounce on any doc or tech who said anything remotely inconsistent or inaccurate. At my appointment, I knew that the uterine lining should be about 8 mm for insemination, though sometimes doctors will still do an IUI if the lining is 6 or 7 mm. The ultrasound revealed that my lining was still paper-thin at 1.6 mm. Meanwhile, the follicle was quite advanced at 14 mm. A "ripe" follicle reaches approximately 22 mm, and follicles grow about 2 mm a day, which meant—quick math—I had at most four days to thicken my lining. Even with supplementation, that was an unlikely prospect.

With the ultrasound complete, the tech quickly herded me out the door, promising, "The doctor will call you shortly to discuss your options." But with those dismal numbers, I already knew my options. I could start taking estrogen immediately, hoping against hope that my lining would catch up with the follicle. It was a long-shot, but once again, pregnancy had only ever been a longshot for me. I wasn't going to give up now. So I moved on to the next step in this intricate dance: ordering sperm for the right day. If the follicle grew as anticipated, I would need sperm early Monday morning. It was already Friday.

As I picked up my phone, a lingering dread crept in, leftover from my last interaction with the sperm bank a few days prior, which had felt only slightly less stressful than wrestling an alligator. *How is it that someone who spends her whole day "helping" people in delicate emotional situations can be so rude?* Anyway, from Ms. Alligator I had learned that I could have my samples couriered to me on Monday for $125, or FedExed on Saturday for $245. This time, a different but equally surly woman answered the phone and explained why neither of those plans would work. The only option was to pick up the samples myself, in Palo Alto, that afternoon. I squeezed her into waiving the same-day processing fee and headed for my car, steeling myself against a seventy-mile drive to the opposite side of the Bay Area, in Friday rush hour traffic. This would take hours.

It wasn't just the traffic that had my blood boiling as I inched my way toward Palo Alto, though. It was past three, o'clock and the doctor still hadn't called me back. Every minute that passed was another minute I could have been thickening my lining with an estrogen prescription. Did this mean she had deemed the lining too thin and the follicle too advanced? Was I slow-rolling myself through a traffic-clogged freeway for no good reason? I was starting to fume.

At five-thirty, the doctor finally called, while I was in my car, driving home, with precious frozen cargo in the back seat. On first beat, the tone of her voice told me the news was bad. She recounted the stats I already knew, then she dropped the bomb, "We obviously already have concerns about your egg quality and quantity. But now I'm concerned about the fact that your lining is not thickening. You might have scarring or some other uterine problem that could entirely prevent pregnancy." I held my breath as she continued a conversation I had not expected. "I would advise that you call off this cycle. If your lining thickens, then I would suggest you move forward with an egg donor cycle. But if your lining is still thin, we will need to do some further testing to figure out why your lining won't thicken."

My brain struggled to decipher her words. I might not be able to carry a baby at all? Even via egg donation? Was she saying I might never get pregnant? "If my lining doesn't thicken, what does that mean?" I stammered. "Will we be able to fix it so I can carry baby?"

"It's hard to say. Most of these types of issues we can fix with minor surgery. But we won't know till after a test cycle," she calmly explained.

I needed to digest this information, but I knew my time on the phone with the doctor was limited, and I still had more questions about this cycle. "Is there any chance my lining could thicken for this cycle? It thickened quite well on estrogen last cycle." Maybe I was in shock, unable to U-turn so quickly, but in that moment I was not ready to give up when I had follicles developing and I had vowed this would be my last attempt with my own eggs.

"I wouldn't advise it, but it's up to you," the doctor said. "There's no harm in continuing."

I tried to gather my wits about me. *Okay, so it's a much longer longshot than I thought.* There would be no medical harm, but I needed to weigh the stress, potential for disappointment, and financial cost. This tug of war between hope and failure was taking a toll on me. But was I more comfortable trying than giving up? I'd gotten this far, and already I had decided this would be my last attempt with my own eggs, no matter what. Miss Leave No Stone Unturned could not walk away until she had tried *everything*. "Okay, I think I need to try."

"Okay, that's fine. Schedule a sono for Monday morning," she said before hanging up.

I was stuck in the car for another hour, trying to get home from the sperm bank, battling late afternoon Bay Area traffic, breaking into tears every few minutes. I was still upset that I'd lost so much time to thicken my lining, but more to the point, I had always assumed egg donation was my choice if I wanted it. I was shocked that it might not be so simple. I assumed I had control over this choice. The realization that yet another door might be closed had me in a terrible panic. My hands sweat profusely as I gripped the steering wheel with all my might, replaying the conversation over and over.

On Monday, when I arrived at the RE's office, the tech painted a hopeful picture. "Your lining has thickened to 4.4 mm from 1.4 in about two days. Quite impressive! And your follicle is about the same size as before. Let me go tell the doctor on duty to see what she says." When she left the room, I felt the sweet relief of her words washing over me. Might this cycle have its miraculous ending after all?

When the tech returned, she informed me that the doctor was happy with the update and instructed me to make an appointment for Tuesday or Wednesday, to keep an eye on the follicle. When I got home, however, my doctor's assistant called with a different story. "The follicle isn't growing, and your lining is still thin. Because the follicle isn't growing, you can stop the estrogen and cancel the cycle," she explained.

What. The. Hell? "I don't get it," I said, recounting what the doctor on duty had told me a mere hour ago.

"Oh yes, that's true," she said, changing her tune. "If you want to continue the estrogen and check the follicle in two to three days, you can."

What? Now I was utterly confused. *How am I supposed to decide what to do when I've been told two completely different stories? Why did the assistant reverse her recommendation so suddenly?* I was losing faith in my fertility clinic. Again. In the end, I reasoned—if you can call it reason—that I'd come this far against their advice, so I needed to soldier on. Checking the lining would put me out another $300, but it was still less than the cost of a vial of sperm.

Two days later, on Wednesday morning, I lay on the exam table, waiting for my third and final ultrasound. I tempered hope by reminding myself that the entire cycle had been fraught with ups and downs. I feebly explained to yet another tech why I was there and what we were hoping to observe. After probing my insides for a moment, she turned the display screen toward me. "There's nothing there," she said. She showed me the right ovary—nothing, then she pointed out a small, insignificant follicle on the left.

Impossible. "The tech on Monday had a really hard time finding my ovary," I explained. "Can you look again?"

For a split second, confusion rippled across her professional neutrality. "There's no evidence of a follicle on either one of your ovaries. Not one about to ovulate or one that has just ovulated. I do see something either on the tip of your ovary or just off to the side.

I can't tell if it's on your ovary or not. It might be on the very tip."
She paused and pushed a call button. "I need a second opinion."

When the second tech arrived, the first gave her my backstory,
and they peered at the ultrasound machine, brows furrowed. After
a mumbled debate, I heard, "We need to ask a doctor."

Enter the third character in the morning's drama, a relatively
young, blonde doctor, whom I had never met before. After briefly
introducing herself, she examined the screen, then told the techs,
as if I weren't in the room, "No, that's not her ovary. You're right.
There is a space between what looks like her ovary and the thing
that looks like a follicle." She glanced my way and pronounced,
"It's a cyst on your fallopian tube, not a follicle."

The room started to spin. I held back tears, took a breath, and
tried to hear my questions through the tornado's din. I didn't want
to seem like an overly emotional, overly reactive basket case, and
yet that's exactly what I felt like.

The doctor explained that cysts were normal. "They can come
and go. No big deal," she said casually oblivious to my mounting
distress. Clearly she wasn't concerned, but I felt defeated. *Now
something else is malfunctioning in my reproductive system?* As the
doc deciphered this latest debacle, I worked hard to maintain my
composure.

She continued, "The other day your ovary and tubes must
have been so close together that we confused the cyst for a follicle, thinking it was on your ovary. Your tubes and ovaries move
around all the time. We can clearly see they are separate now." She
forged on, paying no heed to the fact that her techs had read two
previous sonograms incorrectly, skyrocketing then plummeting
my hopes. "You need to discontinue the estrogen and this IUI.
Take Provera to induce your period and then start an estrogen test
cycle next month." She turned to my chart, flipped through a few
pages, and then continued, "It's time to assess your options. Oral
medications are thinning your lining and not working to get you
to ovulate. After the test cycle, you should move to an egg donor."

"Is that my only option?" I asked.

"You could consider injectable drugs to induce ovulation,

because they give us more options to thicken your lining and produce eggs." This doctor did not mince her words. "It's not medically
recommended, given the fact that you have only one resting follicle
and other poor indicators. But, it is your choice. The chances that
you would get pregnant are incredibly low."

Injectable drugs? I knew I should be asking for more information, but like a boat captain navigating through fog, I had difficulty finding the questions. No matter, the doctor's words were
swirling together—I couldn't decipher her meaning. But the gist
of it I got—using my own eggs was not working, even with drugs
and careful monitoring. Through the fog, a slew of unanswerable
questions emerged: *How bad is this going to get? Is my regular doctor right? Is something wrong with my uterus, preventing the lining
from thickening? Will it prevent pregnancy of any sort—my eggs,
donor eggs, and donor embryos?*

That day I left the exam room in a numb daze. The tech and
the office staff seemed uncharacteristically sweet and conscientious
as I checked out. I went into autopilot, making words come out of
my mouth, handing over my credit card to pay $300 for the scan.

"We'd like you to schedule an appointment with your primary doctor to assess the situation and figure out next steps," the
receptionist said.

Are you kidding me? I'd spent $900 over the past week, to
follow a follicle that was actually a cyst. I'd clocked how many
miles in my car, how much time on the phone, how many hours
in appointments, chasing a conception attempt that had just dissolved on the ultrasound screen? The last thing I wanted to do was
to drive to San Jose, over an hour and a half from my home, to drop
upwards of $300 to meet my primary physician in person.

"She can call me," I grunted.

I was outraged about the money I had spent on unnecessary
scans, and I was upset about the news, but the clear-headed part of
me knew that, really, I was angry with my own body and searching
for someone to blame. So instead of unleashing a torrent of anger,
I reminded myself that everyone involved was doing their best.
I reached deep into my mind to retrieve my mantra, "Nothing

except love makes sense." I repeated it while finishing my transaction. I repeated it as I left the building, walked across the parking lot, climbed into my car, and shut the door. *Nothing except love makes sense. Nothing except love makes sense. Nothing except love makes sense.* Rather than starting the car up, I sat for a moment, tears flooding down my cheeks. This was it, the end of the road. No exit. I was done hoping. Trying to beat the odds was futile. It was time to give up the genetic link to my child. Indeed, I wasn't even sure if my Plan C, a donor egg pregnancy, was possible. The words tumbled out of my mouth, surprising me, "Just give me a baby, and I'll be grateful!" I said out loud. "I don't care how it gets here."

And with that, a deep calm settled over me. The tears stopped. My body relaxed. My jaw unclenched, and my heart softened. I felt myself surrender. The months of anguish over using an egg donor, the incredible struggle to use my own eggs—they dissolved on the spot. I could stop hitting my head against a wall, trying to produce an improbable outcome. In that moment, I felt clear: I just wanted to be a mother. I would do whatever it took, and if I had the honor of bringing life into this world, I would feel blessed.

Despite my clarity, I wanted to connect with Chris for a temperature check. Would he tell me to keep trying? Or would he encourage me to move to egg donor? I texted, "I think it's time to use an egg donor." I paused before pressing send, absorbing the definitive statement. Sharing this newly-accepted truth with Chris felt significant. He'd been guiding me with such love and care for over ten years. He knew me intimately and cared deeply about my well-being. He'd been supporting me every step of this journey to motherhood. He knew how much I wanted a baby. He knew how hard I'd been trying. I took a deep breath and pressed send.

A few moments later, he responded, "Good plan."

My heart sank. *Had I hoped he'd counter my intuition? Had I hoped he'd send words of encouragement? Tell me to have faith and not to give up?* Instead, Chris was affirming my tender truth, meeting me at the crossroads, and coaxing me to move on.

A sense of loss lingered over the next several days, as I continued to research my options. Part of me regretted giving up without allowing my body one more chance to kick out an egg with the proper lining. When doubts arose, trying to derail me from deep knowing, I settled myself by finding the supports of my skeleton and waiting for a deep, calming breath to arise. Almost instantaneously, I'd find "home" again. Regret and doubt would vanish, allowing me to move forward in my research. In my better judgment, I knew I'd never had an optimal IUI because my body wasn't capable of producing that. I didn't need to let the question of genetics eclipse my desire to be a mother. I would love any child I was given the opportunity to raise.

plan C

As promised, my doctor at the fertility clinic called within a few days. "I'm ready to move on to egg donation," I explained. I shuddered internally when I uttered these words, my new reality settling deeper into my psyche. "What are my options?"

"Great. Your chances of success will increase to match that of your donor's age. Your first decision is between fresh and frozen eggs. We have finally perfected the technology for freezing eggs. It's called vitrification, which basically means a flash freeze. It reduces the buildup of crystals in the eggs as they freeze and has very good success rates," my doctor explained.

"Wow, it's amazing that the technology has changed so quickly," I marveled. This was not an option a few years prior, when I'd discussed it with my OB/GYN.

"The advantage to frozen eggs is that you do not have to sync your cycle with the donor, and it's much cheaper. I can have the nurse send you information about it," she offered.

With egg donation, I could expect a normal pregnancy, and any concerns for the health of the baby would be calculated based on the egg donor's age, greatly reducing the risk of Down syndrome or other factors. The physical process was quite straight forward.

For my test cycle I would begin estrogen for two weeks, after which I would have an ultrasound to confirm that my lining would thicken. Then I would have a saline flush to check for polyps and fibroids. If all that checked out, I would inhibit my cycle to prevent ovulation with the drug Lupron and begin estrogen to thicken my lining for the embryo transfer several weeks later. If I decided to use a fresh egg, my cycle would be synched precisely with my donor and she would be undergoing IVF to hyperstimualte her ovaries. As soon as her eggs were ripe, she would be given a trigger shot, and her eggs would be harvested and fertilized. At the same time, I would begin taking progesterone to mimic ovulation and the second half of my cycle. Depending on how the embryos developed, we would plan for a transfer of an embryo into my body three to five days after fertilization. I would continue taking progesterone for the first ten to twelve weeks of my pregnancy, when the placenta would take over progesterone production.

As far as the eggs themselves, I had to choose between frozen or fresh eggs. The cost ranged between $18,000 to $50,000—nausea-inducing numbers that would decimate my savings. Not to mention, I was so frustrated with my fertility clinic I was loath to fork over this kind of cash to them.

I lined up the questions I needed to answer: How soon did I want to start the cycle? Did I want more than one child? What information could I get on the donors? Which options provided Open ID donors? What were the costs and success rates of my different options? Instead of following the instincts of my inner lawyer, obsessively Googling into the wee hours of the morning, I trusted my gut. When I felt the enthusiasm to gather information about an option, I did. When I couldn't muster the energy to research, I let that option fade into the background. Along the way, I kept returning to the fact that frozen eggs had many advantages, the most important to me being the cost. But vitrification was such a new process, and I personally wanted to keep conception as natural as possible by having a fresh egg. There had to be a less expensive way to conceive with a fresh egg. An OB/GYN friend from Chile had mentioned once that egg donation in Chile was much cheaper. I took a break from my research to call her.

Sure enough, she jumped into action immediately, emailing the head of the fertility program in Santiago. Within a few days, I received an email from a doctor, asking for my phenotype and a picture, so they could find a suitable donor who matched my physical characteristics. Matching my looks was not a priority for me. I was more concerned about intelligence, creativity, and feeling an energetic connection to the donor. But at $5500 the price was right, and I had dear friends to stay with in Santiago, so I wanted to make it work. I sent the information and a current photograph, and week or two later I received an email from the doctor: "We found a great donor for you. She matches your phenotype, graduated from college, and teaches kindergarten."

"Great, how tall is she? And, can you tell me anything else about her background?" I emailed back.

A few days I heard back, "No, we can't tell you any other information. She's a good donor."

Apparently there was an inverse relationship between the amount of information provided and the cost of the process. Yes, I wanted to save money, but I needed to see a picture to assess the donor energetically. And I wanted to be able to provide more information about the donor to my child. While a vacation IVF sounded kind of nice, I needed more than Chile could offer. A virtual tour of fertility clinics around the globe revealed that only Panama, South Africa, the Ukraine, and Mexico offered photos. Mexico emerged as my front runner when I found a video interview of a doctor at a clinic in Cancun. His demeanor struck me immediately—caring and concern, a sweetness palpable in the video. For the first time since I had begun this journey, I felt like I'd found a doctor with his heart in the right place. I wasn't naïve enough to think he wasn't concerned about money, but I trusted my instinct. There was something different about him.

Cancun scored another point in the "pro" column because I could stay with Laura at her hotel in Tulum, only two hours from Cancun. She'd still been begging me to come visit. Mexico was singing an intoxicating tune. I filled out preliminary paperwork for two fertility centers in Cancun. Meanwhile, I called Laura to float the idea of an IVF vacation. "It's a fraction of the cost of the US," I explained, "and I only need to be at the clinic for two appointments. The rest of the time I could hang out in Tulum."

"Wait, wait," Laura interrupted. "Are you sure the doctors are reputable?" Having done business in Mexico for the last twenty-five years, Laura was unsure.

"Yes," I assured her. "The doctor of the clinic I am most interested in was trained in Europe, and the program seems legitimate. It's big business these days, so they can't get away with anything shifty."

"Okay," Laura replied skeptically. "As long as you've done some research on it. Of course you can stay with me. It would be my honor to be part of this journey with you."

The puzzle pieces were aligning seamlessly, drawing me toward Mexico.

A few days later, Laura and I spoke again. "I think you should come," she exclaimed. "I did some research on IVF here and you are right, it does seem on the up and up. And what do you think about the idea of going to Mexico City for a few days before arriving in Cancun?"

"Ooohh, I love the idea. I've always wanted to visit Mexico City. How fun!" After a year of struggle and disappointment, I felt joy and playfulness reentering my life. I followed it. "What about going to Cuba for a few days too?" I was giddy with excitement at the thought of traveling, one of my great loves. I yearned for the freedom and novelty.

"I'm in," Laura exclaimed. We burst out laughing. Travel, salsa dancing, warm summer nights—Cancun was speaking my language.

I sensed only one glitch in my Cancun plan: Mexican law required donor anonymity. If by some small chance my donor signed up with Donor Sibling Registry, an independent organization that connects donors and families, then we could find each other, but I needed to accept the likelihood she'd remain anonymous forever.

Research suggests that children born of donors felt it very important to meet their donors, which is why I had chosen an open identity sperm donor. I certainly did not want to harm my child in any way, but in the realm of egg donation, the cost differential was dramatic. Using an open identity egg donor in the US would cost four times as much as the Mexico option. If I'd been making the choice years later from where I sit now, I might have made a different choice. Now, the statistics from frozen eggs cycles have nearly caught up to fresh egg cycles and some frozen egg banks have begun offering Open ID donors. What's more, if I'd realized how much money it would cost to raise a child and enroll in preschool, I might not have balked at the cost of a fresh cycle egg donor in the US. But at the time, preserving those funds to support our family seemed so critical. I would still be my son's biological mother and this felt like a material difference. He would not lack a mother as the result of egg donation in the same way that he would lack a father as a result of sperm donation.

When I first started researching donors, Chris shared his perspective. "Ideally, your child should be able to meet the donor. It's important for a child to satisfy their curiosity about their origins. I can't say what your child will want, but I know life wants to happen."

Choosing to use an anonymous donor was one of the hardest decisions I made in my journey, but I felt like I had no other good options. It felt impossible to go into debt to get pregnant. And, with the advent of places like 23andme and Ancestry.com, I wondered if it was really possible to remain an anonymous donor in the world of genetic testing? This might provide some options for my child to explore his origins. I would register with the Donor Sibling Registry, a site founded to help donors and offspring connect, at my first chance, and cross my fingers that the egg donor would be curious and connect with us at some point in the future. And, if not, I vowed to keep the lines of communication open with my child, and I hoped that my honesty, and good intentions would help my child understand my choice.

For the next two weeks, I considered potential donors from two different clinics in Cancun. Like I had when picking my sperm donor, I would use whichever clinic had the egg donor I wanted. I spent hours with their profiles, though "profile" is probably a generous word. Other than adult pictures, the clinics provided only eye color, hair color, height, weight, age, and the answers to a few questions such as "What are your hobbies?" and "Why do you want to donate?" Most of the answers were less than a sentence long, some in broken English.

After ranking donors, I polled friends. Amazingly almost all of them named the same two donors as their top choices, which just so happened to be my top two as well. One, a Mexican woman in law school, was cute and bright. The other, a Caucasian woman born to French parents in Mexico, shared features similar to mine—cheek bones, eye structure, lips, and nose. Her energy felt uncomplicated, easy.

In a final step, I enlisted Chris. In a Skype chat, I shared my excitement about going to Mexico then launched into my pros and cons for each donor. But Chris interrupted me, "You've already decided which donor to use. You actually know the answer in your body, but your head is getting involved and confusing you again." This old habit—the chattering, worried mind usurping my clarity. I was thankful to have Chris there, once again, to remind me to trust my own knowing. "When I listen to you speak, your voice calms when you talk about one of the donors. Do you know which one it is?"

"No, I'm totally confused," I responded. Mired in the back and forth, I'd lost touch with my wisdom. I took a deep breath to ground myself. I noticed my body making contact with the couch, pulling me into presence. Next I placed the pictures of the egg and sperm donors beside each other on my computer screen and started describing them to Chris. Suddenly I could feel it: the match between the Caucasian donor, the sperm donor, and me.

"I'm getting this overwhelming feeling that it's just simpler with the donor who looks like me. I don't know why but it's less complicated. There's a synergy between the three of us." As I uttered these words, my body settled more deeply into the couch, my jaw relaxed and my mind stopped chattering.

"Yes," Chris said. "Listen to that. I believe she is the one you have already chosen. I don't believe you could go wrong with either, but I do feel a resonance between you and her." This donor had been the top pick amongst the majority of my friends as well.

I could feel the truth, in my body and in Chris's words. She was my donor. I was so relieved to have made what felt like the most significant decision of my life, choosing the woman who would pass her genes to my child in my place. A wave of gratitude washed over me. This woman was providing her eggs to me. She was putting her own body, and potentially her future fertility, at risk for my sake. If our roles were reversed, I doubt I would have been willing to undergo IVF or to give away my own genetics. Yet here I was, receiving this beautiful gift. I wished I could hug the donor, thank her for giving me the greatest gift she could ever give someone—a child. Of course, I'd never be able to communicate with her directly, and what words would convey the depth of my appreciation anyway? Months ago, I had balked at the idea of spending money on an egg donor, but in this moment the transaction felt nothing like incurring an unwanted expense. It felt like receiving an enormously generous gift.

As soon as I hung up with Chris, I called the sperm bank to arrange my sperm vials' Mexican vacation. Honestly, I was dreading the call. The first time I had spoken to the sperm bank about my Mexico plans the representative had told me, unequivocally, "We do not ship to Mexico." He explained, "We rarely get our shipping tanks back from Mexico, so we stopped doing it."

I never knew what I would get when I called the sperm bank. Sometimes I'd connect with helpful people willing to jump through hoops for me; other times, I'd find an obstructionist on the other end of the line, unwilling to help with the sometimes complicated logistics of sperm shipment. This time? Well, off the bat I detected a note of annoyance in the representative's voice. Did I just roll into her bad day, or was she simply a customer hater? *Here we go . . .* I shared the briefest possible version of my backstory, then—hoping my enthusiasm would be contagious—explained how excited I was to have found a way to address their concerns about losing or damaging their tanks, "I found a private courier who will come pick up the sperm vials, put them in his *own* tank and hand-carry them onto a plane to Mexico."

"We will not ship to Mexico," the representative explained.

"I know," I said. "But you are not shipping to Mexico. I'm getting a private courier. You just need to fill out the necessary paperwork and the courier will come get my vials and put them in his tank."

"Since we don't ship to Mexico, we can't fill out your paperwork or release your sperm to this courier."

What? My frustration started to mount. "This is absurd. I own this sperm. *You* are not shipping the sperm. I know you do not want to risk getting your tanks cut open. But the courier will not use your tank. You just need to issue the paperwork."

"We will not issue the paperwork," she replied in a bitchy tone.

My attorney self stepped up. She was not making sense; I was going to point out the ridiculousness and possibly illegality of her claim. "Let me get this straight," I said, "You are going to hold my property hostage?"

"We will not issue the paperwork," she repeated.

"I'd like to speak to a supervisor," I spit out, holding back a wall of tears.

"I *am* a supervisor," she said cattily.

I felt a surge of rage course through my body, but just before I completely lost it, I realized no matter what the conversation it wouldn't end well. This woman was a dead end. Instead of spurting out all sorts of profanities and insults, I needed to calm myself before continuing. Maybe I'd get a kinder, more flexible representative if I called back later? At that same moment, my doorbell rang. Through my glass front door, I saw Jane and Leonardo, friends from Chile, arriving for a week-long visit. I carefully said, "Thanks. I'm going to call back later," and I hung up.

an unlikely offer

As I pulled Jane and Leonardo into a group hug, I was suddenly overcome by wracking sobs.

"What happened?" Jane asked. "Are you okay?"

When I failed to respond, they held me closer and let my wordless tears flow until I could speak. I collapsed at the bottom of the stairs in the entryway and sputtered, "The sperm bank is refusing to ship my sperm to Mexico, where I am planning to do an egg donation cycle. They're also refusing to release my samples to a private courier for transport. It's ridiculous. It means I don't have a sperm donor to use."

"Don't they have sperm donors in Mexico?" Jane asked cautiously.

"They do, but they provide so little information it's unsettling. There are no pictures, just an Excel spreadsheet with hair, eye color, height, weight, and ethnicity. I can't face telling my child the only information I have about his father is a single line in an Excel spreadsheet!"

At that moment, Jane burst out, "We'll donate! Leonardo will give you his sperm. Won't we?" she said, nudging Leonardo in the arm.

"Yes, yes, of course," he said, though his hesitation to speak signaled to me that he wasn't as sure as his wife.

"You want this so badly," Jane said. "How could we deny you

the opportunity to have a child? You've worked so hard for this. We won't let a lack of sperm stand in the way."

Torrents of love poured into the room, connecting us all. I felt my chest flutter as my heart opened to receive their gift. "But you realize this means Leonardo would have another child in the world?" I said cautiously, sure this would cause them to renege their offer.

"So? How cool! Another child in this world related to us but I don't have to raise it? What a blessing!" Jane joked.

"C'mon, it's settled," Leonardo said as he patted me on the back reassuringly. "What do we have to do? Surely my age is a problem, though." Leonardo was about my age, I guessed about forty-two. Contrary to previous beliefs that sperm did not degrade with age, new research was suggesting that older sperm might contribute to birth defects and autism.

I immediately dismissed his concerns. "Well, no, you're not too old. Men much older than you have children all the time. Plus, we can have your sperm analyzed for genetic abnormalities and motility. You could come to Mexico for a few days while I'm there and donate a sample that would be used in the IVF procedure. I'll happily pay for your tickets." How wonderful would it be to have my friends with me in Mexico.

"Great! Done!" they exclaimed, looking at each other reassuringly.

I'd always known these friends had my back if anything ever were to happen to me, but this—offering Leonardo as a donor— stretched beyond my imagination. I was still choking back tears, but now because of the beauty of their offer, not my frustration with the sperm bank. "Well, it would be amazing. But seriously, I insist that you guys think about this for twenty-four hours. It's a huge decision. Your children would have a half-sibling?"

They blew me off again, insisting it was decided.

Our day continued in South American fashion, lounging on my deck, soaking in the gorgeous, 80-degree weather. We sipped white wine in the middle of the afternoon, while Leonardo opened a vast pile of packages he'd had mailed to my house; items that were cheaper in the US than Chile. This was our tradition—Christmas in summer with wine lunch.

I marveled that our interactions were so natural. We had nothing in particular to do except enjoy each other's company. Leonardo opened his packages, Jane read a local San Francisco magazine, and I futzed around, intermittently taking care of things and relaxing. We came together to laugh and share a funny thought. We were all so at home together.

As afternoon rolled into evening, I wondered about the impact of using a known donor. Up to this point, my journey had been so scientific and methodical—carefully-timed inseminations, sterile doctor's offices, vials of frozen sperm. Would this act of love shift something, allowing me to get pregnant?

At a random moment, walking upstairs, the beauty and love in my friends' offer hit me. My eyes welled up, and I felt my chest tingling, breaking open at my heart center. Leonardo, Jane, and I had been close for years. We'd fantasized about buying property in some remote part of Chile, raising our children and retiring there together. Already Leonardo was a dedicated father, and though I didn't expect or want him to be a father figure, I imagined meeting up with Leonardo and Jane for holidays, growing closer to their entire extended family. I was already friends with his sister, and I loved his mother as well. Jane and I had formed a sister-like bond the minute we met over a decade ago. I couldn't think of another couple with whom I felt equally close to both halves of the equation. My heart knew this could work. I wanted to run downstairs and shower my friends with gratitude. But before I could act on that impulse, embarrassment took over. I quickly cleared my tears away and composed myself, checking a mirror to make sure it didn't look like I'd been crying.

My head, on the other hand, begged me to listen to reason. Hadn't I rejected the idea of a known sperm donor because it seemed too complicated? Sure, using Leonardo's sperm might provide me a family support system, or at least a sense of community. It might help me to feel connected to someone on my journey. But I could also sense confusion and messiness on my behalf. Here I was saying to myself that Leonardo would be a donor, not a dad, but at the same time I was fantasizing growing closer to Leonardo, Jane, and their extended family, even hoping Leonardo's sister and mother might look upon my child as a relative.

Leonardo, Jane, and I continued lazing around together, laughing, drinking wine, playing games. But eventually the conversation turned back to their offer. My lawyer mind wanted to talk logistics. "We can sign a contract that says I can't ask for child support and that you, in return, are releasing paternity rights," I said, thinking this would put their minds at ease about any scary legal parts of our arrangement. But I saw them both pause, the first hint of hesitation as the impact of what they'd offered started to register. A wave of disappointment washed over me, and I realized in that moment how much I truly wanted this. Nonetheless, I was heartened to see them thinking more carefully about the ramifications of their decision.

A few moments later, Leonardo caught sight of Jane trying to insert her phone's new SIM card into the memory slot. "Ouff, nooooo, that's not how you do it." He said it jokingly, lovingly, but his disapproval was clear. This triggered a cascade of worries. Leonardo, as lovely as he was, was also a relentlessly opinionated Virgo. In fact, it was a running joke between the three of us—when Leonardo disagreed, he'd grunt, "Ouff!" This had become part of our parlance, "Don't ouff me, Leonardo," or "Is that going to get an ouff?" In our friendship, I could make light of his "ouffs," but what would it be like to have Leonardo tied to me and my child? As the donor, would he be able to withhold his opinions? What if I wanted to put my child in a public school and Leonardo didn't think it was good enough? Would he pressure me to enroll the child in a school I couldn't afford? How would I respond to his hints of disapproval? How many parenting decisions would become unnecessarily complicated?

Many single moms by choice run into this dilemma eventually, and I wondered now whether knowing my donor—and the prospect of my child knowing the donor—was more important than any potential emotional messiness or legal debacles? Known-donor complications could range from minor disagreements straining a friendship to donors suing for partial custody against a mother's will. In the risk-benefit analysis, some women forgo the benefits to avoid the risks, while others take a leap of faith. Now it was my turn to face the dilemma.

I had heard and read many beautiful stories about known-donor relationships, but these were tempered by horror stories about donors who decided they wanted more involvement with the child. The laws surrounding the use of a known donor are murky at best. I already knew this. Leonardo could sign a contract releasing his paternity rights, but if conflicts arose, there were no guarantees that the court would enforce the contract, especially if Leonardo had any contact with my child that could be interpreted as a father-like role. Even if we signed clear contracts, emotions don't fit in neat legal boxes. I could not predict how I would feel about Leonardo and Jane's involvement or lack thereof, and I assumed the same would be true for them as well. Even if we avoided a legal battle, we might create an unnecessary strain on our relationships. Was I willing to take that risk?

Later in the day, when Jane and I were alone in my living room, I asked, "Are you sure this is something you want to do? You do realize what it means—Leonardo would be the biological father, even though he would not be involved?" I paused to make sure my words were registering. When I saw her tracking with me, I continued, "Your children would have a half-sibling. How would you explain that to them? And, conversely, I'd have no genetic link to the child whatsoever."

"Yeah," she said, shifting her eyes to the floor. "It is a lot to think about, huh? It's basically like giving a child up for adoption."

"Yes," I responded, my heart sinking with the realization this might not happen. We had all sobered up, literally and figuratively. Doubt and caution were creeping in like clouds on the horizon.

For the next few days, though it was the only thing I was thinking about as we wandered the city, soaking up all the Bay Area had to offer, none of us brought up the donor idea. Even though it was Leonardo's sperm involved, I preferred to discuss it with Jane, and I took my chance after dinner one night, as Leonardo slept in the back of the car.

"What have you guys been thinking?" I asked.

"Leonardo doesn't think he could ever relinquish control," Jane responded, as she looked out the window across the Bay to the city lights. "He'd always feel responsible."

"Yes, I can feel that it's the sticking point." I said. I recounted my moment of clarity about getting "ouffed."

"Yeah, you don't want to subject yourself to getting 'ouffed' all the time. Trust me," she said, and we burst into laughter. "That doesn't mean we won't do it, though. I think we've just realized that it's much more complicated than we initially thought. But if push comes to shove, we want you to have a child, and we would never deny you that. So, we will do it if you need us too, but I think you have to exhaust all other options first."

"I totally get it. On the one hand, having Leonardo as the donor feels so amazing. I know that he is a dedicated, loving father. It would make me feel so comfortable, and it would be so fun to visit in summers and share the upbringing of my child. But I can see that it could get complicated, too. Not to say that it would be horrible, but definitely much more complicated." I knew there were no guarantees—it could bring us closer or it could drive a wedge in our friendship. "And I haven't exhausted all options yet," I continued. "I still might be able to get the sperm bank to comply. Or figure something else out."

With that, I knew Leonardo wasn't the guy. I'd been wooed by the idea, but I needed the simplicity of an unknown donor. It was the first week of May. My egg donor cycle was set for mid-July. My mission was clear. If there was a way to ship sperm into Mexico, I'd find it.

the sperm challenge

The prospects looked grim. The patient coordinator here in the US, the clinic itself, the message boards I consulted, they all agreed: shipping sperm to Mexico would be prohibitively expensive. I ignored them and soldiered on, but the stress was keeping me up at night. One early morning, after another fitful night's sleep, I got out of bed to do a Tibetan Puja for Wind Horse—the remover of obstacles. It felt like a long shot to call on some remote Tibetan god, but at this point I didn't know what else to do. I could put on my lawyer hat at any moment, but first I would turn to the esoteric.

At this point, my plans for conception had been scrambled and reset so many times, I knew that I could deal with anything. Deep inside, I could trust that I'd be okay, no matter what. But, jeez, how many more obstacles did I need to face? How many more lessons would I have to learn on this journey to become a mother? This lesson I had already learned: when I notice myself beating my head against the wall trying to make something happen, it's time to take a step back and reassess. In those moments I ask myself, am I trying to push forward something that simply doesn't want to unfold? Well, was I? Should I give up trying to go to Mexico and instead pay four times as much to seek an egg donor in the US? Technically, I had the $40K. Was I being too stingy? Too stubborn? Should I reconsider my options in the US?

Aside from the sperm shipment, my Mexico plans had fallen into place beautifully, and I felt comforted and supported by all aspects of the plan. My gut liked the Mexico plan, and I had learned to trust this "gut instinct" knowing. So rather than scrap the whole plan, I decided to push forward, for now. I resolved to raise hell if the sperm bank continued to block my ability to send my sperm to Mexico. I'd found one employee who said she'd regularly worked with my courier. But the day after she had promised to help me, she started a three-week vacation. A few days later, when I'd called to set things in motion, I was notified that my case "was being escalated." The bank was now refusing to sign any paperwork to release my sperm to the courier. "You have to wait until the president of the company decides," the employee on the phone explained.

Incensed, I got ready to unleash the lawyer. If they would not release my sperm, I would seek a full refund, and I would slam them with online reviews everywhere I could. As I saw it, I owned the sperm and should have been able to do whatever I pleased with it. It was not illegal to ship sperm to Mexico. The sperm bank admitted that it regularly released sperm to this same courier for shipment to other countries, and it even FedExed directly to other countries. The sperm bank's guarantee and liability ended once the tank left their offices, so why did they care what happened afterward? Further, I had taken on responsibility for obtaining all the necessary permits and arranged for my courier to use his own tank so theirs would not be damaged. On what grounds was the sperm bank refusing to release my sperm to me? I suspected there was some other underlying issue or policy at play, though I never figured it out.

After a few more heated discussions, the bank informed me that they would grant me a special dispensation and complete the necessary forms for me to get my sperm shipped via the private courier. I was still livid that I even needed a special dispensation, but I decided to cut my losses and move forward with the courier. "I just need the health permits from the governing agencies of the releasing clinic and a letter from the receiving clinic stating that they are willing to accept the samples," the courier said. "And I need one to two weeks lead time to coordinate my schedule and book travel."

After easily securing the health permits, I set to work procuring a letter from the Mexican clinic. Thinking that I had made it through all the hoops, I relaxed. But a few days later, the clinic messaged, "We need to get a permit from the Mexican government. We've submitted the paperwork, so it should only be about fifteen to twenty-one days before the permit is issued."

"But the courier has said he's gotten samples into Mexico before with just a letter from the clinic," I pushed back.

"Okay," the clinic responded. "If he thinks it's okay, then you can ship them without the permit. We will write the letter. Please send us a sample letter so we know what to write."

Excited, I emailed the courier to tell him to go ahead, but now he had changed his tune, "If the clinic in Mexico says we need a permit, then let's wait for the permit."

Ugh. Knocked into limbo again. How many times would this happen? This was absurd. I was ready to throw a tantrum like the toddler I was hoping to raise, but instead I took a breath and agreed to wait the estimated fifteen days for the fertility clinic's permit.

Given my luck so far, I suppose it shouldn't have surprised me that fifteen days passed without word from the clinic. A week after I sent them a follow-up email, they responded, "We need another fifteen to twenty-one days. No one in the state of Quintana Roo, where Cancun is located, has ever applied for this permit before. But don't worry, Sarah, we are doing everything we can." *Right. Don't worry. Sure. No problem.*

Well, at least I had scheduled my egg donor cycle in mid-July, well in advance. But I wanted my sperm to reach Mexico before I boarded a plane in late-June to vacation in Mexico City and Cuba with Laura. It was only late-May, so I tried to remain calm and grounded. However, twenty days later the clinic informed me, "We still don't have an answer. But we anticipate that it will take another twenty days. We are trying our best to help you. But don't worry, if your sperm samples aren't here in time, you can just use one of our donors."

The mention of their sperm donors made me itchy. Under no circumstances would I use their donors, and at this point, I didn't have another twenty days. So I emailed the private courier, asking him to book the flights and travel without the permit if necessary.

"No, let's wait for the permits. I won't book flights until we have the permit," he refused.

Are you *kidding* me? How many more barriers would I meet? How high would I have to climb? I tried a few more emails. "Can you please send me the language of the letter you've used in the past to get your samples into Mexico, so I can have the clinic draft the letter? I'm not comfortable waiting for the permit."

No response.

With only two weeks left before I departed for Mexico City, I went full-on MacGyver, devising wild and whacky back-up plans that surprised even me. I could schedule to pick up my sperm samples in Palo Alto, just as I had done many times before. Then I could speed to the FedEx office to ship them to a friend in San Diego, then jump on a plane to meet my samples there. From San Diego, I'd drive across the border into Tijuana. Of course, I wouldn't get stopped at the border. Of course, no one would search my car, finding a suspicious nitrogen tank. In fact, a friend had assured me, "I will go with you. If you need anything smuggled, I'm your girl. I've taken so many questionable things across that border. I don't get rattled or scared. I'm coming!" Once across the border, I would find a FedEx office in Ensenada and ship the sperm to Cancun, preventing the tank from traveling through customs. Of course I might need some permits in Ensenada, but I felt confident that if I provided the health permits of the releasing clinic, and a letter from the receiving clinic, I'd be able to get it through FedEx. All I needed to do was add some suspenseful soundtrack music, and I'd be good.

Okay, maybe not. So my backup plan was to reenlist Jane and Leonardo. But my gut didn't like this plan, and my enthusiasm for it had cooled. No part of me wanted to risk changing our friendship forever, so I devised plan three: find a donor in Mexico with the help of my friend Laura. I called her to talk prospects. "I still don't have my sperm samples in Mexico," I explained tentatively, knowing she'd been skeptical of my shipment plans all along. "Do you know anyone I could use? I am desperate, and I'll pay."

Laura had lived in Mexico a long time and had a small hotel's worth of employees—she had to know *someone*, right? Maybe we could set up a live version of *The Dating Game*, except we'd have to call it *The Mating Game*. Her guests could vote to select my donor. See? Fun for all! Though Laura and I had a good laugh considering potential candidates, underneath it all I felt saddened by the prospect. I had put so much care into picking the right donor, and now this desperation to find anyone willing? It still seemed better than choosing a line off the clinic's Excel spreadsheet, but neither were what I had envisioned for my baby.

My final plan? Take the tank to Mexico City myself, stopping through Cancun to drop it off at the clinic on my way to Cuba. Of course, I'd have to get the tank through customs myself. While I felt fairly confident in my powers of persuasion and flirtation, the stakes were too high, and doubted I could rely on the private courier to share any tips. He was still refusing to provide even a sample letter for the clinic, so why he would give up the goods to help me get through customs?

With only ten days left before my fight to Mexico City, I enlisted Chris's advice. Should I keep waiting for the permit or try another route? "Sounds like you're at a dead end," he said. "You need a new plan. After people have messed with you for a while, you need to recognize it's not going to happen and take a new course. What about finding another sperm bank which *will* ship to Mexico for you?"

I was dumbfounded. Why hadn't I thought about this easy solution? Here I'd been plotting potential crimes and other outrageous scenarios, when all I needed to do was find a willing sperm bank. I'd been so attached to my donor and the money I'd paid for the vials that this simple idea had never crossed my mind. Within an hour, I found a sperm bank willing to ship vials of sperm at a moment's notice via FedEx. I called to confirm their policies. "We ship over fifty percent of our vials overseas," the representative said cheerily. "We have a person dedicated to navigating customs issues. We can get your samples there within a few days for about $350."

Really? It was *that* easy? Though I was not looking forward to picking yet another donor, I was elated to find the clinic. Hopefully I'd learned a thing or two through my first two donor searches, and I could apply those lessons now.

Luckily, I would have some time alone with Chris while traveling back from a retreat in Southern California, so I asked him if he would review profiles with me. Well, *begged* might be a better word for it. In the Southwest terminal of the Burbank airport, we opened up my laptop and commenced sperm shopping.

This bank provided adult pictures, which made it much easier to get an intuitive hit, so we went straight to the photos first, often without even reading their information. Chris was very enthusiastic about the first donor we looked at. "He'll work," he said with a little chuckle. I knew he meant it, but the idea of stopping there unsettled me. On my insistence, we continued to open more profiles. After about five or six donors, Chris said, "I have a feeling it's the first one. But let's keep looking."

By the time we boarded the plane, we had a list of about twenty possible donors. "Go home tonight and rank your top three to five donors," Chris advised. "I'll look at them tomorrow and help you pick the final donor."

Because I needed to turn over every single stone before I could decide, I continued to consider even more profiles when I got home. But my process was completely different this time. Finally, I was able to trust that I did have enough insight and intuition to make a good choice. I didn't analyze endlessly the written details of each profile. I looked at the pictures, and I took a brief glance at the written essays and physical characteristics. Every once in a while, I would dive deeper into the profiles for hobbies, indications about IQ, and well-rounded personalities. But instead of obsessing over whether the donor seemed creative and smart, spoke a second language or played a musical instrument, I simply looked for health and vitality. I focused on my felt sense. Would I feel comfortable showing this donor's profile to my child?

Whenever I paused to rank or re-rank the donors, the first donor remained in pole position. Chris had known this immediately, but I had a different process for reaching my knowing place. Considering all possibilities calmed me down enough to hear my intuition. Yes, Chris had an amazing ability to see things, but working with him, I had learned that I too had the ability to discern what was best for me. I sent my ranked list to Chris for a final review and he confirmed, "The first donor is the one. None of the others work." With this affirmation, I breathed a sigh of relief. In fact, this new donor felt so perfect to me that I wondered how I'd ever been attached to my previous donor at all.

As soon as I awoke on Monday, I called the new sperm bank and paid for two vials of sperm. The bank directed me to provide the receiving clinic's exact address and the name of a contact person at the clinic. With this information, they would be able to ship out my sperm samples the same day. It was that easy. I'd been tooling around with the previous sperm bank for nearly two months, losing sleep because of the anxiety, while this simple solution had waited for me to notice it.

On Wednesday, I pulled the trigger and asked the sperm bank to FedEx that day. I didn't bother to double-check whether the fertility clinic in Cancun needed anything else, because I didn't want to know. On Friday, the sperm bank called to let me know that my vials had arrived in Cancun, but were stuck at the FedEx Customs office. "Don't worry, Sarah," the overseas liaison from the sperm bank assured me. "Sometimes shipping to Mexico is tricky. There might be some extra fees, but they will get through." So I waited through the weekend on tenterhooks, and on Monday morning, I received notice from the clinic, "We finally got your permit and were able to get the samples," it said.

The permit the clinic filed for months ago—it miraculously came through on the day my vials showed up in customs? What's the word for "simultaneously dubious and grateful"? Whatever it is, that's how I felt. I finally had sperm samples in Mexico, proving yet again that where there is a will there is a way.

the shot

While I was mapping my sperm's circuitous route to Cancun, I also was starting the protocol to sync my cycle with my donor's, which began—ironically—with taking birth control for a few weeks. Next up, I needed to give myself a shot of Lupron, so I could take estrogen with no concerns about ovulating. My Lupron shot was scheduled for the morning I would fly to Montana for Qigong retreat. I'd been so preoccupied by my sperm challenge and preparing for my trip, arranging for dog care and house sitters, that I didn't so much as look at the Lupron box, which I had gotten from a friend in Mexico, until the night before I needed to take the shot. I figured it would be fairly straightforward, until I discovered the instructions were in Spanish.

Considering my meticulous nature, it seems strange I would drop the ball on preparing for such an important step in the protocol. Then again, when it comes to making a baby, there are so many important steps to take, so many decisions to make, so many variables to consider and arrange just so—it makes sense I'd lose track of a detail here or there. With traditional conception, nature makes the decisions and calls the shots. But when a woman decides to conceive using assisted reproductive technology, she's essentially taking over as general contractor on the project of building a human. Well, if it was inevitable I'd overlook a detail, at least I overlooked a relatively simple one.

Not to worry, I thought. *I'll ask Joanna. She's a doctor and she's been through IVF*. I texted her, "Can you coach me through how to give a Lupron shot?"

"I have no idea," she responded. "I think you should ask your clinic."

It was now 10:00 P.M., and I was leaving at 8:30 A.M. the next morning. How would I figure it out before then? I fired off emails to my contacts at the clinic in Mexico and to all my doctor and nurse friends, hoping someone would get back to me in time. I tried rereading "the protocol" sent to me by the clinic, but it didn't say if the shot should be administered subcutaneously, meaning just under the skin of my belly, or intramuscularly, meaning jabbing the needle several inches into my butt.

I tossed and turned all night long, dreaming of needles. Ass or stomach—either one sounded gross. By 5:30 A.M., I could no longer sleep, so I jumped out of bed to check my email, hoping the three-hour time difference would mean someone at the clinic had responded. The patient coordinator had emailed. She was a far cry from medically trained, but I didn't care. At this point I'd take any guidance I could get, which was, according to her, "intramuscular would be preferable." *Great*. So, I consulted my other medical expert, Google, for intramuscular injection training. Ta da! Up popped exactly the short course I needed. I had just two concerns: (1) I needed to avoid the sciatic nerve and major arteries, (2) The thought of stabbing myself in my own ass with a two-inch needle set my heart racing and my hands shaking.

I rushed around all morning writing emails about the dog care schedule, showering, and packing. At 8:15, I had five minutes left to administer the shot before my ride to the airport arrived. At that moment, my roommate emerged into the kitchen, innocent to the act about to take place. As a chiropractor, she'd have the anatomy skills I needed. I pounced on her, pleading for help. However, as a chiropractor, she'd never given a shot. "I'll help," she said, "but I'm pretty squeamish. I might have to look away."

Good enough. I fumbled the packet out of the refrigerator and set all the items and the directions on the island. I took a deep breath and told myself now was not the time to rush. Together we deciphered the confusing pictures included in the Spanish directions. Then we mixed up the Lupron ingredients, and I pulled down my pants, leaning over the kitchen island. Who would have imagined *this* would become part of our tenant-landlord agreement? My roommate plunged the needle into my ass.

"That stings," I gasped.

"It's only about halfway in," she said. "It stopped."

Before I could make a joke about my rock-hard gluts, she aspirated the needle, and it sunk in deeper. "It's only about three quarters of the way in," she reported. "Do you want me to push it in farther?"

I cringed at the thought. "That's good enough," I said through clenched teeth.

She pressed the syringe plunger, and I felt cool liquid seep into my flesh.

Before I could wonder about the success of our awkward endeavor, my ride arrived at the door. As we drove to the airport, the absurdity of the situation became clear: I had just asked my roommate to plunge a needle in my ass. Typically this honor would go to one's husband or partner, but not so for me. I suspected this was only the beginning of asking random people for help. They don't say "it takes a village" for nothing.

vacation, baby

My friend Laura and I arrived in Cancun on Sunday, July 7. After ten jam-packed days in Mexico City and Havana, we checked into a business hotel a few blocks away from the clinic. I would have an appointment at the clinic the next day, then I would take a taxi to Laura's hotel in Tulum until my transfer a week later.

Laura and I ate at a health food restaurant, gorging ourselves on vegetables, which were sparse while we were in Cuba, and then we headed back to the hotel. While traveling, I'd clocked about five to seven hours of sleep a night, I'd taken two hours of dance classes each day, and I'd downed several *cafecitos*, and plenty of rum and mezcal. I was both enlivened from my trip—the laughter, the vibrant colors, the art, the dancing—and beyond exhausted. Now here I was in a comfortable bed, nestled in soft, clean white sheets and perfect pillows, ready to catch up on sleep.

But I tossed and turned all night, my mind racing. In Cuba, I'd been completely detached from communication with the outside world. Back on Mexican soil, I'd expected to find an email from the fertility clinic updating me about my egg donor's response to the medications. Instead, radio silence. My mind clicked into worst-case-scenario overdrive: the donor doesn't have many eggs; my lining won't be thick enough because I'd opted to use oral estrogen—which I'd already had—instead of purchasing the recommended estrogen patches; my cervix will be tightly closed, making it impossible to insert the catheter without jostling the embryo or damaging my lining; my sperm samples will have died or worse yet, they won't use the right sperm. What if they didn't label it properly? The list continued.

The next morning, I nervously got dressed, grabbed a quick bite to eat, and met the prearranged taxi driver, who delivered me to the clinic promptly at 9:30 A.M. Emma, a tall, beautiful Hispanic woman, greeted me, inviting me into her office. Her big smile and sparkling eyes made me feel instantly at home. The clinic was gorgeous, with sparkling white marble floors and walls conveying a vibe both modern and (thank goodness) sanitary.

Emma and I got right down to business. So far I had not paid the Mexican clinic any money at all, even though my donor had started the process weeks prior. "Do you have a copy of the agreement?" Emma asked me. "I can't find a copy." The agreement, so sparse it hardly could be called an agreement in the first place, was now missing? Clearly we were not in the United States, where contracts and money always come first.

Relax and trust, I kept telling myself. *Remember, the first moment you found this clinic, your heart immediately said yes.* Though their style was relaxed compared to the US, this clinic had always come through. If I was going to allow this to be an enjoyable process, I was going to need to trust it rather than nit-picking every move.

After paying, I was led into an exam room, where a young, attractive doctor met me and introduced himself. *This is not the doctor I saw in the videos,* I thought. But before panic could take hold, I told myself it seemed reasonable that an assistant doctor would conduct a routine exam to check the thickness of my lining.

The doctor initiated a conversation about the procedure, but before he could finish, I bombarded him with questions about my donor's progress. "How is she doing?" I asked.

He consulted my donor's file. "Great," he said. "She has at least fifteen follicles maturing. Everything looks great."

Yes! This was the information I'd been waiting for—fifteen follicles meant plenty of eggs, upping the likelihood that the clinic would produce enough viable embryos for me to get pregnant. In short, the donor's ovaries just gave Project Baby the green light. Actually, fifteen green lights.

Next the nurse then showed me to a five-star-worthy private restroom adjacent to the most luxurious exam table I'd ever seen. And that's saying something, because at this point, I was nothing if not a connoisseur of exam tables. In fact, it wasn't even a table. It was more like an ultramodern reclining chair, featuring padded stirrups. I undressed from the waist down and waited for my exam.

Turns out the doctor on duty who had startled me with his unfamiliarity not only had a kind bedside manner during my exam, but also the ability to perform a pain-free mock transfer. Also, he delivered more good news: my uterine lining was at 9.43 mm. Neither too thick, nor too thin, but like Baby Bear's bed: just right. Everything was on track: my uterus, my cervix, my donor, and the doctor had won my confidence.

I was escorted back out of the treatment room, where Emma reviewed my protocol with me and sold me the progesterone I would need to start taking on Wednesday. Then she called a taxi, which delivered me to the bus stop for Tulum. I bought my ticket and a snack, and I was on my way. Relieved beyond measure, I slept for most of the two-hour trip on the comfortably air conditioned bus.

I arrived in Tulum, greeted by Laura who was eager to hear how my day at the clinic had gone. I ate a platter of fish tacos and guacamole at the beachside restaurant and then retreated to my room to rest more. I spent the next few days swimming in the warm crystal blue waters, lounging in the sun, doing Qigong on my private deck, and taking long walks up the beach. Paradise.

On Wednesday, two hours up the coast, my future baby was being conceived in a petri dish, without me. Not exactly the scenario I had imagined as a dreamy, baby-obsessed child, but miraculous in its own way. The clinic had already warned me I wouldn't get any details about the fertilized embryos until the following morning, so when Laura suggested a day trip to Valladolid, a colonial town about an hour away, I agreed.

The market, the convent, a high-end perfumery, the traditional Yucatan restaurant with a woman making tortillas right there in the middle of the dining room—I was happy for these distractions, though I spent many moments sending love to both my donors and thinking about the kind of essence I wanted to attract—sweet, gentle, uncomplicated, an old soul, wise, and balanced.

When we returned to the hotel, I took a two-hour walk on the beach alone, attempting to send intentions and thoughts to my baby (or babies, rather) germinating in that petri dish up the coast. Yet, my mind kept drifting to a cute boy, Miguel, whom I had met in Tulum two years ago during a salsa dancing vacation at Laura's hotel. The first time we met, he stopped dead in his tracks and told me how beautiful I was, then he scurried over to our group leader to ask about me. We flirted and danced for an entire week. He too did Qigong, so we woke up early one morning to share our Qigong practices with each other. It seemed inevitable that we would kiss, but we never did. By chance he had been in Mexico City while we were there, and we all met up to go dancing. "*Mi salsaera*," he exclaimed, embracing me in a huge hug. And just like that, the flirtation that had begun two years ago kicked into gear. The dance chemistry was amazing, but still no kiss.

Now, as I walked along the beach trying to send my baby love, my thoughts kept drifting into fantasies about a fling with Miguel— how we'd go out dancing then walk home along the beach together. How we'd stop to have a swim in the bathtub-warm water, under the full moon, watching a giant turtle lay her eggs on the beach . . . *Stop.* I'd tell myself. *Your baby is being conceived today.* I would return to my original intention, sending love to my future child, imploring my teachers and helpers to bless this baby. Already I'd enlisted Chris and all my Qigong friends to do some special practice today, to help make this baby a reality, blessing it with lots of good juju. And here I was in la-la land, fantasizing about a cute boy? I managed to shift my fantasies slightly: I imagined myself at this beach with my baby and other friends who had children. We'd hire a nanny so we could go out dancing. I'd meet up with Miguel and walk hand in hand down the beach to the outdoor salsa venue. In the morning, we'd wake up and take both our children to the beach.

Yeah, this wasn't working. I tried a different tactic: mantra. That would occupy my mind and bring goodness to my baby. The first mantra that popped into my head was Dzamla Za, the Tibetan god of prosperity, abundance, and wealth. I focused on abundant growth and conception, though it seemed a little off track. I switched to White Tara, the mother of all and grantor of wishes. I strolled down the beach, singing her mantra and begging her to protect this life and grant me a baby. After twenty minutes of White Tara, I switched to the mantra for my Qigong lineage. I asked, or begged, rather, for a baby, promising to raise my child in the Qigong lineage. And more importantly, promising to be good to my child, to provide support and structure, while allowing for my child to have his or her own identity and personality.

The next morning I awoke early, checking for news about the embryos and finding none. I kept myself occupied swimming, reading, and writing, but underneath the relaxation a niggling anxiety vibrated. Occasionally I'd follow its lead to the restaurant where I could get Wi-Fi and check for updates. Around noon, the update finally arrived: twenty-two eggs or oocytes were retrieved, twenty of which were mature, and seventeen of which fertilized into zygotes. I had no idea how many embryos would make it to day five, but with those numbers it felt safe to say I would have many chances to get pregnant, even if it didn't work the first time. With that news, the anxiety buzz silenced, and I headed back to my beach chair to soak up more sun.

Later that afternoon, I again took a walk down the beach to do mantra for the little cells. It struck me how much life had come into being, on my account, that may end up stunted in frozen limbo, never coming to fruition. I had no idea what that meant morally, but in reverence to what had occurred on my behalf and just in case, I prayed for forgiveness for any harm I had done or any suffering I may have caused. *I am so grateful for the abundance you have provided me, and I apologize for any harm I have caused. Thank you for bringing so much life into being on my account. I am sorry if there is any suffering. Please know, however, that any harm caused had good intentions. I am deeply committed to this baby. I will take amazing care of it, providing support and encouragement but trying my hardest to let his or her nature be expressed. I will try my hardest to help this little being know his or her perfection. As to the brothers and sisters that I don't gestate, I will seek guidance on what is best for them: donation to another single woman or couple, long-term freezing, or eventual termination. Again, I apologize and ask for forgiveness, but I assure you it was done with the best of intentions.* As my prayer released into the atmosphere, my heart settled, relieved and ready to receive any gift life might bring.

On Friday morning, I received another update from the clinic: we had only lost one; sixteen zygotes. "So, we will do a day three transfer at 12:30 tomorrow," the email concluded. What? If there were so many zygotes, why were they rushing to do the transfer? I shot off an email to the patient coordinator, "Why the day three transfer? I thought it was better to wait until day five? Can you tell me what factors they are basing their decision upon?" Then I jumped online to research: "Day three vs. day five transfer when using egg donors."

The results were mixed, which likely means that no one actually knows. From what I gleaned waiting until day five meant the zygotes would have progressed into blastocysts, a ball of seventy to a hundred cells comprised of two different types of cells, making it more likely any unviable contenders would be eliminated naturally. Also, in old-fashioned sexual reproduction, the fertilized egg would not travel into the uterus until day five, so transferring on day five more closely mimics the natural progression. Day three, on the other hand, had been the industry standard until recently, but only because the technology necessary for day five transfers hadn't developed yet. Some people argued that getting the specimen into your body as soon as possible had its advantages, but there seemed to be a consensus that day five was preferable in a sophisticated lab, with a considerable number of zygotes. My gut was telling me to aim for day five, but I sent the doctor an email anyway. His response: "Don't worry, Sarah. You can do a day five transfer."

Immediately, I peppered him with questions. "What? Wait a minute. What does the embryologist think? What factors is this being based upon?"

Again, the response: "Don't worry, Sarah. Day five is fine. Your transfer will be on Monday at 11 A.M. You need to arrive at 10:30 A.M."

After a few more emails back and forth with Emma and the embryologist, I finally reached the doctor on the phone. "You got the wrong email. Your embryos are doing really well, so we should wait till day five," he explained a little too casually.

The wrong email? What would have happened if I hadn't asked about a day five transfer? I took a breath, reminding myself to relax and trust. I *had* asked the question, and that was all that mattered. The lack of information, the doctor's laisse faire attitude—clearly it took a certain kind of person to do this procedure abroad, and I was learning to be that person, learning to let go.

Speaking of letting go, as long as my beloved embryos were in a petri dish two hours away, I could have some fun: caffeine, alcohol, swimming, staying up late—you name it. And I had already named it. Months ago, I'd decided I wanted one last fling before embarking on motherhood. I couldn't imagine dating while pregnant, or in the first few years of my child's life, for that matter. I wanted one last hoorah, and time was running out. As luck would have it, Miguel was scheduled to arrive on Sunday. My last pre-motherhood fling, the day before transfer: flirting, dancing on the beach, big laughs, and some kissing fun.

the blue light

iguel arrived Sunday, as planned, with his adorable four-year-old son, and his sister. As Miguel and I watched his son play in the water together, he asked me, "Do you have children?"

"No, but I want them," I responded guiltily, not wanting to explain.

That night we danced at a huge Cuban salsa festival, including a *Rueda*, meaning wheel in Spanish. In this Salsa equivalent of square dancing, someone calls out the moves and the dancers, wheeling around each other, constantly change partners. Over forty-five couples had joined the dance in three thrilling and beautiful nested circles on the beach.

At the end of the evening, with his son in bed, Miguel came back to my cabana and we made out. It felt innocent and sweet to kiss and cuddle all night long, just what I needed. Before we fell asleep, I explained that I'd be leaving early in the morning. "*Necessito ir a Cancun mañana muy temprano,*" I pieced together with my small amount of Spanish.

"No. *Yo, te puedo manejar a la playa,* you can get a bus from there," he offered.

"*Quiero un taxi,*" I explained. There was no way I was trusting a bus to get me to the most important appointment of my life.

"*Un taxi es muy caro.* I take you to bus station. *Conoces* ADO, the bus company?"

"No, *un taxi es mejor para mi,*" I explained. I needed the comfort, ease, and predictability of a taxi driver whom Laura knew taking me to Cancun. How could I explain to Miguel why I would spend at least $150 for a taxi to Cancun? Since our conversations always took place in a broken mishmash of English and Spanish, I feigned incomprehension. I leaned over and kissed him to say enough talking for now. He dropped the subject.

At seven-thirty the next morning, I whispered, "*Adios, Miguel. Hasta pronto.*"

"*Si, mi amor,*" he said through a sleepy haze. "It was beautiful to see you."

With that I headed off to Cancun, leaving one life behind for another. I hoped.

After a nearly two-hour car ride, when I arrived in Cancun, I needed to pee, badly. The restroom was occupied, so I perused a Vogue México, waiting for my turn. But a nurse came to get me. In a combination of broken English and Spanish she said, "Come with me, Sarah. I'm going to show you to a room where you can wait. Do you need water?" she asked, filling two cups of water and lead me down the hall. "Are you nervous?"

"No, not really. Mainly excited," I said.

"Drink this and do *not* pee pee," she cautioned.

"But, I already need to pee," I tried to explain.

"*No!* No pee pee," she warned in her thick accent, waving her index finger at me.

Since we'd done a mock transfer at my previous appointment, I understood that they needed my bladder full to position my cervix and uterus. But I was already desperate for the bathroom, and my procedure wasn't scheduled for another hour and a half. So I snuck into the restroom and took a half pee. Thank god for years of pelvic floor work. Then I dutifully drank the water provided;

changed into a hospital gown, hair cover, and booties; and lay down. The nurse returned to the room, "Here's a remote control, Sarah. You can watch TV."

I had planned to use this time intentionally, to recite some mantra or call in my baby, but my mind kept returning to the events of the night before. My time with Miguel had been so lovely, a nice distraction from my pregnancy worries. But it felt strange to be so unfocused now that the moment was near. I hoped my support team back home was doing some practice for me, because, with only a few hours of sleep, I was worthless. I tried to drag my mind to recite some mantra, "*om mani padmi hung*," but the moan of my aching bladder drowned it out. I needed something to distract me from the water balloon sloshing in my lower regions. The TV was playing *Grey's Anatomy* in English, and in that moment Meredith told Derek she was expecting their baby. There it was: my ticket to Distractionville.

Forty-five minutes later, I was fit to burst when the doctor came in to discuss my embryos—the same one who had performed my mock transfer. My heart sank. I'd been told the head doctor, the one from the video, would be doing the transfer. But then I remembered this doctor's masterful and painless transfer, and I relaxed. "You have seven embryos left, Sarah. We will transfer two, freeze two and continue to watch three of them to see if they develop enough to warrant freezing. Here's a picture of the two embryos we will transfer."

"Two embryos?" I almost jumped out of the bed. "No, I only want to transfer one. The success rates are very high, aren't they? If I transfer two, it's likely I could end up with twins, correct?"

"Okay, Sarah, don't worry. That's fine. Yes, the success rates are high with blastocysts, so it's fine if we only transfer one."

"Which one do we transfer? How do I choose?" I stared at the sheet of paper with the pictures of the two embryos, and my mind started racing. *How do I choose? Eeny, meeny, miny, moe? What if I pick the wrong one? Should I transfer two, just to avoid the decision?* But my senses quickly returned to me. I did not want twins under any circumstances. When people conceive the old-fashioned way, nature makes all these choices for them. I decided to relieve myself of the responsibility. This time, I'd let the powers that be do their thing.

After a pause the doctor continued, "Let's let the embryologist decide between the two strongest."

"Yes," I agreed. *Perfect. Let the scientist choose.*

After thirty minutes that felt like an eternity, the nurse came in wheeling a stretcher that looked like a prop from *Grey's Anatomy*. I climbed on and was rolled into a sterile, cavernous room. The largest lights I had ever seen hung from the ceiling, on giant moveable arms. When the doctor entered a few moments later, he showed me a TV mounted on the wall, where I'd be able to watch the action on a split screen, one showing the ultrasound of my uterine cavity, the other featuring the embryologist's petri dish.

"Sarah, are you comfortable?" the doctor asked, pushing on my bladder.

"No, I have to pee quite badly."

"Well, Sarah, I need to catheterize you and drain your bladder a little. It's too full for the transfer. But don't worry."

I tried to interrupt him to ask if I could simply get up and pee a tiny bit, but he was blazing forward. He showed me the catheter and began threading a tube, about a small pinky finger wide, up my urethra. I winced and started to cry almost immediately.

"Don't worry, Sarah," the doctor assured me again. Was he serious? It hurt like hell and felt incredibly unnatural. All my effort to hold my pee led to this? Apparently "don't worry" was a catch-all phrase for this doc and the staff. I felt my pelvic area go into spasm, and I tried to calm the shaking.

"I'm sorry, Sarah. I know it's uncomfortable, but now we are ready for the transfer." He gestured toward one half of the TV screen. "Here you can see the embryologist suck the embryo out of the petri dish and into the catheter." I watched as a thin, needle-like object entered the image of the petri dish. "Look, Sarah, over here. Do you see that little grey dot? That is your embryo." My potential future baby looked like a spec vacuumed up off some space-age carpet.

"Okay, now, Sarah, we are going to insert the embryo into your uterus."

I willed myself to move past the pain of the catheterization, so I could be fully present in this moment. I closed my eyes, took a deep breath, and called upon all my helpers. *I will love and care for this baby like no other. I want this baby more than I've ever wanted anything.* Every step I had taken on this fertility journey was culminating right now. I pleaded and begged. As I did this, behind my closed eyelids a wash of blue light came over me.

"Look here on this ultrasound. Do you see that little bubble that just appeared in your uterus?" the doctor gently spoke, pulling me out of my prayer and the wash of blue light that had enveloped my field of vision. I could see it only vaguely. "Now look over here again," the doctor said directing my attention back to the white screen. "They are going to empty the catheter and make sure the embryo isn't there. Then we know for sure it's in you."

I watched the first screen again as the embryologist flushed the catheter. Several big black bubbles came across the screen and then disappeared. The faint grey bubble did not appear, at least that's what the doctor told me, and since the image on the screen looked to me like nothing more than a grainy, black-and-white landscape, I decided to trust his assessment.

The nurse wheeled me back to the same waiting room I'd been in before and advised, "Don't get up for at least ten minutes," then disappeared out of the room. I tried to remain still for another ten minutes, still desperate to pee. *What did that blue light mean?* I wondered. *Blue is often the color of healing and health. The Medicine Buddha in Tibetan lore is blue. Or had I just welcomed a baby boy into my uterus?* It seemed ridiculously cliché: *Blue light for a boy!* But I couldn't shake the sensation.

Within the promised ten minutes, the doctor arrived with a picture of the embryo in my uterus. Embryo number nine. "Take it easy for the next week. No swimming in the ocean or pool, no running, stay out of the sun, and no sexual intercourse," the doctor advised. Then he shook my hand, "Good Luck, Sarah. Keep us posted," and left me alone in the room.

Back in Tulum, Laura and I dug into a huge bowl of chips and guacamole as I recounted the details of the transfer, grateful to share such a monumental experience with a friend. "By the way," I mentioned, "I need to administer a shot of progesterone in my butt tonight. Can you help me?"

Laura busted out laughing, "No way. I am so squeamish. I will pass out if I even see a needle. Sorry."

We laughed so hard tears formed in our eyes, but mine were tinged with sadness. Suddenly, I felt so tired of doing everything by myself. Mostly, I felt perfectly happy walking this path to motherhood on my own, but at times like these, my aloneness stung. The sting was about my situation, not about Laura. I knew this wouldn't be the last time I called for help and no one came.

Laura didn't give up though. "Let's ask Juan Carlos," she suggested. Juan Carlos was the manager of Laura's restaurant. He was sweet and caring and someone I would have been attracted to if we'd been closer in age. "He'll do it. Someone can cover for him at the restaurant so he can take a break and help you."

No way was I going to ask a near stranger, and the manager of Laura's restaurant no less, to stick a needle in my bare ass. "Uh, no thanks," I insisted. "I'll do it myself, but will you stand outside my door so you can call for help if I need it?"

"Sure," she agreed. "But even standing outside knowing you are giving yourself a shot might make me faint."

I eyed her with a skeptical glance, "C'mon, don't be ridiculous. I'm the one giving myself a shot."

After watching a few videos to understand exactly where and how to shoot up, I retreated to my room while Laura sat just outside on a hammock. Actually I was feeling pretty brave as I pulled down my pants, leaned over my bed, reached around with the syringe in my hand . . . and then I stopped. There is something incredibly unnatural about stabbing oneself with a two-inch needle. With the needle poised above my skin, I knew one quick jab would do it, but I just couldn't get my arm to lunge forward. I took a deep breath. *Remember why you are doing this.* And with that, I stabbed the needle into my ass. I pushed the plunger and pulled the needle out, and popped my head out the door. "I did it!" I called to Laura. "I feel like such a badass!" I exclaimed.

Laura ran over and slapped me a high five. "That's great! I can't believe it!" she said.

Wasn't this what motherhood was all about? Overcoming my fears and getting it done? If so, I'd just passed my first test. I was ready.

disbelief

*T*wo days later, I reluctantly left the paradise of Tulum and flew home to wait for that magic day when I'd take a pregnancy blood test. I was no stranger to the two-week wait by this point, but it felt different this time. I knew I had a real shot at getting pregnant, and I felt confident—wrongly or rightly—that eventually I would get pregnant with donor eggs. The desperation of previous attempts at conception had faded, and I was at peace.

A few days later, I attended Chris's monthly Qigong workshop. Upon entering the classroom, I avoided the other students and walked straight up to Chris. Attempting to act casual, I made feeble small talk before launching into my burning question, "So how do you think my project worked? Was it successful?" Maybe it was unfair to ask, but I couldn't help myself.

"You don't feel it?" Chris asked, hands tucked in the pockets of his hoodie. He shrugged, "You are completely different."

"No, I don't think so," I responded. "I haven't noticed anything. I got sick with a stomach bug the day after the transfer, and I've been sleeping ever since I traveled home."

"Your energy signature and chemistry are completely different," he explained. "You have the signature of a woman preparing to be a mother. You dropped a bunch of stuff. It's like your body said, 'Right, I'm going to be a mother, there's no time to mess around,' and so it dumped a whole pile of unhealthy information. You look really good."

"Really?" I marveled in disbelief. "The only thing I can tell is that, if I am pregnant, I think it's a boy. Every time I try to tune into it as if it's a girl, I feel lost and don't find anything. But when I link to it as if it's a boy, I find something quite distinct. And, for some reason, from the very first moment after the transfer, I immediately thought 'boy.' And I haven't been able to shake that feeling." I paused briefly, "I'm curious if you have a read on it?"

After a short pause, Chris smiled and said, "Oh, yeah. I do think it is a boy. You are washed in quite masculine energy. A very willful boy, actually. He might be challenging for you, but also very good for you. As long as you don't squash his essential personality, he'll be very strong and potent."

I knew Chris was about to leave town for about three months, and just the thought stirred up insecurity. "You can't leave without treating me," I begged.

"You are actually doing really well. You don't need my help at all. You are on automatic pilot now. It's been done. You just need to sit back and relax. Try to have the attitude of sunbathing while you are pregnant," Chris advised.

I couldn't hear it. "Yeah, but I took such bad care of myself on vacation. I was up late drinking, dancing, eating wheat and dairy, even had a fling, you name it." I was convinced I needed some serious clean-up, plus I wanted help clearing the pain and violation of the catheterization.

"Okay, you can have a session," Chris assured me. "But as far as I can see, you are actually doing better than I have ever seen you. Whatever you did on vacation suited you. It feels like you were living true to your nature and that did you wonders."

By about ten days after transfer, curiosity got the best of me, and I bought a box of home pregnancy tests. The clinic had urged me to wait until the lab test fifteen days after transfer, but by my math, fifteen days after transfer was akin to twenty days after ovulation and about nineteen after fertilization. Most home pregnancy tests claimed to detect pregnancy fourteen days after ovulation, so maybe I could get some answers early? Call it willful indulgence, but I couldn't help myself.

The very first test was positive—sort of. My test showed two lines, indicating positive, but the telltale second line was supposed to appear within three minutes. Mine took over ten minutes, and even then it was so faint I could barely make it out. Was I hallucinating? Was this wishful thinking? Only one way to find out! I started testing several times a day. Over time the second line was growing darker, but it always took about ten minutes to show up. So I consulted my good friend Google, seeking insight into test brands, false positives, and faint lines.

According to the two-week wait forums, this pregnancy test did not generate false positives and often results took ten minutes to appear. Still, to be sure, I analyzed several images of pee sticks submitted to the forums by hopeful women. Yes, there are whole websites dedicated to women submitting pictures of their pee stick tests so complete strangers can assess if they're pregnant. And yes, there I was at midnight, comparing my sticks to the pages and pages submitted. My conclusion? I should trust my lines. Unless you were given an HCG trigger shot to induce ovulation, which I wasn't, a second line, no matter how faint meant pregnancy.

Since I'd been burned before, I wasn't ready to make that pronouncement conclusively—not even to myself. I continued taking multiple home pregnancy tests a day, adding a second brand into the mix for good measure. On the third day, an undeniably clear second line broke through my defenses. Yes indeed, I was *pregnant*.

On July 26th, I took the official blood test at the lab. Despite my positive home tests, I remained anxious awaiting the results, knowing anything could happen in the early days of pregnancy.

At five o'clock, I was at a restaurant overlooking Lake Merritt, enjoying appetizers with a friend when an email notification lit up my phone: my doctor had posted the results. I asked her forgiveness, while I frantically signed into the secure website to read the results: HCG 119. *What does that mean?* I did the math. When I got my false result, they said my HCG was 461, consistent with two and a half weeks pregnant. When I took this test, I was just under two-weeks pregnant, and since HCG is supposed to double every forty-eight hours, 119 sounded like a very reasonable number. I did it! *Finally,* I had slain the infertility monsters and passed through the castle gate. But my stay in the pregnancy kingdom was anything but secure.

Forty-eight hours later, according to protocol, I repeated the blood test. By late afternoon, the results still hadn't been posted. I started pacing my house, trying to figure out what to do to keep myself busy, while my mind spun the worst-case scenario wheel. What if something was wrong—like the HCG number hadn't doubled? Or what if my HCG had skyrocketed, indicating twins? Either scenario would trigger the doctor to call me personally, rather than posting my results online. Maybe she simply hadn't had time to call and break the news?

What had Chris said? Pregnancy should feel like sunbathing? So why couldn't I sit back and enjoy being pregnant? Apparently at each landmark, a new concern would arise. Would I *ever* relax? Staying calm was the best thing I could do for the baby, but that was way easier said than done.

The next morning, no longer able to wait, I called the lab. The answering service refused to release the results. "There are notes here that I don't understand," she explained. "I'll have the doctor call you. It will probably be about fifteen to twenty minutes." Was this protocol? Or had something gone wrong? Maybe this woman simply had no authority to release my results? At a loss, I spent the next hour trying to keep busy and calm. After making myself a healthy smoothie, I stood in my living room and did some Qigong practice, but I was easily distracted, intermittently stopping to check email, go to the bathroom, and pet my dogs.

An agonizing hour later, the phone finally rang. "Your HCG is 277," the on-call doctor said. I started trying to do math, but I was so nervous that simple arithmetic evaded me. The doctor continued, "Your HCG has increased by 60 percent, which is still considered

normal. But let me calculate it." If her math was correct, sixty percent was not good. I knew it. "Ah, yes. Sorry my math was wrong"
the doctor said, "it's more than doubled. That's great. Are you having
spotting or anything? I wasn't clear why you called?"

"No, I feel normal. I was just tearing my hair out waiting for
this result. I got worried when I didn't hear back. I'm sorry I bothered
you." Though in all honesty I wasn't sorry I bothered her—I couldn't
believe that the doctors hadn't posted my results or called me sooner.
They *must* know women are agonizing over these numbers.

"Everything looks good," the doctor reassured me. "Now, you
just need to schedule your first ultrasound for about seven to eight
weeks."

I breathed a long sigh of relief. Surely now I could relax. My
HCG was normal. I was officially pregnant.

gathering support

I can't say I ever stopped worrying, but my pregnancy progressed relatively smoothly. Spared morning sickness, I remained mobile and active even though I often experienced shortness of breath. Talking too fast or even walking up one flight of stairs would leave me completely winded. I still managed to walk my dogs almost daily, but now it looked more like slow meandering. Of course, I was hit with waves of exhaustion unlike anything I could ever imagine, and I experienced some physical pain on and off throughout, but, considering I was growing a human, I took these discomforts in stride. My twenty-week ultrasound confirmed that I was, in fact, having a baby boy.

While the physical realm remained relatively manageable in the beginning, as my pregnancy progressed it seemed hell bent on testing my feelings about support, or lack thereof. I suppose it made sense that I would be hyperaware of the topic as I sat on the brink of bringing a small child into the world alone. Pregnancy itself—with or without a partner—leaves many women feeling inherently vulnerable. Not only was it physically harder to move around, but I felt vigilant about protecting the life I was carrying inside. However, understanding my sensitivity didn't alleviate my anxiety that I wouldn't have the support I needed. A cascade of physical ailments raised this concern to fever pitch.

It began with a series of intense migraines that incapacitated me for days in a row. After my roommate helped me find a new high-tech pillow, the headaches went away. But a few months later, a bout of sciatica, triggered by a death-defying act—attempting to put on my shoe—flared up so severely I could barely walk. To make matters worse, one night while flipping around in bed, trying to find a comfortable sleep position, I woke to find my arm completely numb. I sat there in the dark for several minutes, shaking my hand and arm, trying to regain feeling. But the numbness and tingling persisted. I was no stranger to this sensation—it was exactly like the pain that knocked me out of my legal career. The symptoms worsened by the day, numbing all my fingers and then both my hands. My mind started to run wild, worrying about the long-term effects of reduced blood flow and impinged nerves. Already I had suffered permanent nerve damage from the original injury, what would pregnancy do to me? Flustered by flashbacks of the years I'd spent in chronic pain, I called Chris. I was falling down the rabbit hole, and I needed to get a grip. On the way to his house, I wondered what I would have done these past years—and what I would do—without his bedrock of support.

As I laid on the table for my session, Chris assured me, "You've done all the work. You have great biomechanics. And your system is incredibly refined and sensitive. When you are off, you need to be adjusted only a hair. You don't need anything dramatic. All you really need is one good breath to fix it and regain your sense of home." Chris showed me the connections between the affected parts of my body—small of the back, between the shoulder blades, sternum, and hands. He slowly and gently worked each area of the body as if to say, "It's okay, you are safe." Sometimes he just touched an area, waiting until a breath would come. Other times he made fine adjustments. As each area let go, I spontaneously inhaled a big, cleansing breath and slowly exhaled. The knot unraveled. "So," Chris asked when he was done, "Do you see how to get out of this next time?"

I hesitated to say yes. If I did, would he agree to treat me next time? The work was so subtle that I worried about whether I truly understood the connections Chris had just pointed out. Would I really be able to help myself next time? I didn't trust yet my ability to support myself, and Chris was about to leave for Bali.

"And, if you are in trouble, you can call me. I will have my cell with me," he said, unleashing a sense of calm over me. In that moment I realized how much of my stress—and even the resulting pain—derived from my sense that I didn't feel supported. In all likelihood, I would never bother Chris on vacation in Bali, but knowing I could was all it took for me to find confidence in my ability to support myself. The ground returned beneath me and the uneasiness dissipated.

As if he could hear my thoughts, Chris suggested, "You need a new mantra! How about 'It's no big deal?' Lots of things might be difficult during pregnancy, but it's important not to get too stressed. Keep repeating to yourself, 'It's no big deal.'"

Oh, right—I was supposed to treat pregnancy like sunbathing. I took a breath, imagining that I was laying on my back deck in the warm sun, and my body relaxed from deep inside. Yes, I could do this. As long as I could separate the fear surrounding my condition from the pain, I could simply focus on the sensations. The sensations themselves were no fun—my arms throbbed, I had a constant tingling in every single finger and barely any feeling in a few fingers. Yet the sensations were bearable if I stopped worrying about what they meant and when they would go away. When I could stay present to what was actually happening, instead of imagining what could happen, I felt secure and grounded. I knew I could handle it.

Over the next few days, weeks, and months, I continued to experience bizarre bouts of pain. But Chris was right, if I did an incredibly subtle movement and waited for a big breath to arrive, I could reset my body and resolve the bulk of my pain. I felt safe knowing that I could help myself. Once I felt adept at this process, I was able to bring it to my students, who also found great benefit from this subtle approach.

~

Pregnancy offered me one last support-seeking tour through my family of origin as well. As the baby grew and my body slowed, my list of things to do took on epic proportions. One night, on the phone with my sister, I expressed the overwhelm. "I've got to get the nursery ready, buy and install a car seat, and finish as many house chores as possible, but some days I feel like I can barely move." Honestly, I was hoping my sister would offer to help, so maybe my tone was leaning toward melodrama, but a moment later my body resoundingly agreed. When I tried to stand up from the couch, a stabbing pain shot through my system, so severe that I yelped. "I can't walk," I choked back sobs. "I'm in so much pain." To my amazement, my sister did not offer to help. As I hung up the phone, sadness overtook me. I would need to seek support somewhere else.

I should have known my parents were the wrong way to turn. Still, most women I knew embarking on single motherhood had family support through either hands-on or financial help, so I guess I got caught up hoping for the same. A few weeks before Christmas, I called my folks and described my situation—the physical pain, the ever-lengthening list of tasks. I asked, "Would you guys be willing to come a few days early to help me with some things?"

My mother barked, "No, do not ask us to help you." I nearly fell over in shock. "We cannot help you. We are old and can barely finish the things we need to get done. It puts too much strain on us."

I wanted to explain that they could help with activities that were not physically taxing, that might actually be fun, like picking out the paint color for the nursery, but I decided to save my breath. When I stepped back, I could understand their position. Both my parents were struggling with decreasing mobility and wavering memories. They too felt overwhelmed. I wished they had the capacity at least to offer emotional and mental support, but who was I kidding? They'd never had that capacity. Nothing—not a pregnant daughter, not a new grandchild—could grant them abilities they lacked. At that moment, I could have spiraled deeper into panic about how I would survive without my parents. In reality, however, nothing had changed. I'd been navigating life without their support for years.

Well, at least I knew where they stood. In this position of absolute clarity, I felt both fearful and calm. How many times had I observed friends lamenting a lack of support from their husbands or parents after their children were born? One thing that had always struck me was that it was the hope that led to the dissatisfaction. That gap between expectation and reality caused most of the suffering. When it came to my parents, I now had complete certainty that they would not help me, so there was no fuel for disappointment. But where my biological family fell short, I had developed a family of my own choosing—friends, colleagues, teachers, and mentors. The support of this chosen family was never more evident than at my baby blessing—my version of a baby shower—organized and hosted by my friends Joanie and Collette.

On the day of the blessing, I arrived at Collette's house to find a beautiful banquet of food, a baby onesie decorating station, and about forty of my closest friends. My sister even drove up from Santa Cruz with a palpable desire to make the day special. After everyone had enjoyed the food and company, we began the baby blessing. We all nestled into Collette's living room. Annette, a natural poet, opened with a poem she had written for my son. Tears streamed down my face as I took in her message of hope and encouragement. My friends continued taking turns sharing songs, memories, kudos, sage advice, and reflections on the liberation our generation had achieved, making it possible for a woman to have a baby alone. I may not have had conventional support—I did not have a husband or doting parents—but I had this room full of loving, supportive friends I could call on for relief.

Of course, there was no getting around the fact that I would be the lone person handling late night feedings, tending to a sick child, and providing the everyday care for my child. I could have fixated on this aloneness, but instead I let it affirm a deeper knowing that I had cultivated through years of Qigong and Feldenkrais practice: *I am supported.* As Chris had said more times than I could count, "If you truly learn how to rest on the supports of your skeleton, you will experience a visceral feeling of support, which is more important than anything else. If you have trouble recognizing support, you can learn to recognize it as a felt experience first. If you constantly feel unstable in your own body, you will struggle to feel stable in life. You will continually seek it." I had come to believe in this foundation of physical support as paramount to my mental health. The mind-body connection I experienced in the first days of my Feldenkrais training had integrated into all aspects of my life and work. I was intimately familiar with the internal feeling of safety and security, and so I called upon it to help me. When I took time to balance on my skeleton and find my supports, I knew in the depth of my being that I was going to be okay, no matter what.

More importantly, I had learned that following anxiety, doubt, or any other emotion for that matter was a choice. During meditation in a Qigong class, I heard a familiar soundtrack playing in my mind: *You aren't doing this meditation right. In fact, you are terrible at meditation.* Noticing the thoughts, I took a moment to ground myself. I felt my sit bones in the chair, ensured that my weight was dropping down evenly through my legs and feet, and allowed my body to melt onto the supportive structure of my skeleton. At that moment, a visual picture of two alternate paths appeared. On the first path, I could indulge these critical thoughts, adding more juice to them and allowing my meditation to derail. On the second path, I could stop those thoughts, recognizing that doubt was my habit—a self-manufactured choice, not a true representation of what was actually transpiring. This was a revolutionary concept that applied not just to meditation, but to all areas of my life. Up until that point, when doubt or anxiety had arisen I had received it as an accurate message, but now I recognized that I had the choice to walk away when it whispered its enticing invitation. When the anxiety about whether I would get enough support called my name, I knew it was a diversion. I didn't need to seek support outside of myself, I needed to trust in my own visceral support. I knew I would land on my feet no matter what. I had proven that to myself countless times on this journey already. Parenting alone might be difficult, tricky, even exhausting, but I would make it.

What's more, I had the support of the intangible. Support with a capital S. I'd developed this faith over the years in my Qigong practice. I can't actually point to any one experience that proved its existence, yet when I reflected on the most troubling times in my life, I could see that things always had a way of working themselves out. Someone or something seemed to be looking out for me, keeping me safe, protecting me from calamity. Though my road to pregnancy had seemed unfairly challenging at times, from a distance I could see something had been watching out for me, guiding me. As alone as I may have felt at times, I knew I was not alone.

facing motherhood

I n my fourth month of pregnancy, I decided to visit a new spiritual teacher that I had heard about for years, named Gangaji. My recently divorced friend, Michael, a father of two, joined me there. We sat in the third row awaiting her entrance. I was incredibly tired after attending a fellow single mom's birth the night before, but I was on a high having witnessed that miracle for the first time. I was listening intently to a story Michael was telling me about parenting, when the room slowly became quiet. Gangaji would be arriving soon. Meditation began.

As I sat with my eyes closed, an immensely bright light emerged. I opened my eyes to see Gangaji walking across the stage, her radiant blonde hair accented by loose, white clothing, her presence filling the room like a cool mountain breeze. She did not speak other than to invite us to sit in silence with her.

Sensations waved through my body as I sat in meditation, most notably a clear sense of the baby's vastness, a direct link to the Vast Perfection. I smiled, luxuriating in this beautiful feeling, as Gangaji began to speak, "Whether it is the first time you have come to see me or one of many, many times, something brought you here. You are seeking something. That seeking is for a home-coming. A desire for oneness." I felt myself melt a little more at the truth of her words.

After a brief talk, she invited audience members to ask questions. A woman, probably in her fifties or sixties, walked up to the stage and sat next to Gangaji. I could see the light from Gangaji radiate off the woman who sat fidgeting with her scarf as she spoke, making the brightness of Gangaji even more apparent. The woman took few moments to breathe and settle herself. "I am a mother of three and a grandmother. But I don't know how to reconcile motherhood and my effort to be a good person." As she burst into tears she managed to spit out, "I wasn't a good enough mother. There are so many things I regret." Her suffering was palpable.

"Oh, my dear," Gangaji reassured. "Neither was I. I could have been a much better mother." The people in the audience, including me, started to laugh. "And I'm sure all mothers could say the same thing."

The woman in the chair looked a bit startled, but she began to laugh a little through her tears.

"So what's the problem?" asked Gangaji jokingly. "We all have things in our life we could have done better. And there is earnest pain about these acts. Can you feel where that pain is in your body now?"

"Yes," the woman replied, as she brought her hands to her heart. "It's right here."

"Can you sit with that? Feel that?" She paused a few moments. "And what happens after sitting with that for a few moments?"

"There starts to be space," the woman replied.

"Yes, space! And a lightness too?" She coaxed. "I don't want to spiritualize your pain away. Your pain is real. But what our teachers have given us is a method of inquiry. So, as you sit with that pain, can you just be with it without trying to fix it, change it, excuse, it, indulge it, ignore it, or spiritualize it?"

Those words, 'indulge it,' caught my attention. If I've been triggered, I can spend hours, even days indulging my story—the fear, the anxiety, the injustice. Instead, could I simply sit with the pain? How many times in the past two years had I indulged in stories—worst case scenarios, fears, or even hopes that hurt me? Chris always encouraged us to allow the pain to be present, but to let go of the story and the bigger meaning we wanted to attach to it.

"The thing is," Gangaji continued, "we all have the feeling of not being good enough. Anyone of us can insert something into the blank. I wish I'd been a better . . . mother, father, daughter, teacher, wife, student, friend. This pain may never go away. But by simply accepting it and being with it you can find space and light around the pain. Beyond that, you can recognize that what you are actually seeking is oneness. All this pain of not being good enough is a red herring from the real pain you feel of not realizing your oneness with perfection. That is the real pain."

When Gangaji listed off the infinite number of things we wish we'd been better at, it hit me like a lightning bolt. Motherhood would stir up every last corner of pain around feeling not good enough. On top of judging myself, and questioning my capacity as a mother, I'd be judged by others. I'd be confronted with it on a day to day basis.

I had a taste of that judgement a few weeks ago when I'd been complaining about my physical pain to my friend Genevieve. "Do you think you should be teaching while you are pregnant? You're just in so much pain," she remarked. "Do you think that is good for your students?" Now it wasn't just my internal dialogue, someone had spoken one of my greatest fears. A part of me knew that my students were learning from me even though I had slowed down considerably, but being called into question by a friend catapulted me into a frenzy of doubt. In the height of my distress, I'd sought out Chris for counsel.

"Ha, are you kidding me?" Chris remarked. "Do you know how many people have opinions of me and the way I should teach Qigong? If I worried about them I wouldn't get out of bed in the morning. Instead, from a place of clarity, I try to understand what might be true about what they are saying and then I move on. Most of what people will say about you is their own projection. Don't take it on."

"But how do I continue to be friends with them if they have bad opinions of me?" I asked.

"Pay attention to how they actually treat you," Chris encouraged. "If someone treats you well, that's all that truly matters. Let them have their opinions."

It was of course an obvious statement, and yet I knew that the most prosaic wisdom was the hardest to live by. Like the trite sayings printed on tea bags, the advice is cheap, but to take it on and make it one's own, that's something. This was an important lesson, one that would serve me well to remember.

I knew from my mother friends that, for whatever reason, complete strangers feel justified in judging others' parenting. But I also knew that, like this mother sitting in front of Gangaji, I would be my own worst critic. I had never thought about my self-judgment as a red herring for the deeper pain of being disconnected from my own perfection. Just as I had come to see doubt as a conscious choice, now I could see that self-criticism was also a choice and more importantly a call to return home to myself and my essence.

As I sat, bathed in the light of Gangaji, I realized my work had just begun. As I contemplated becoming a shepherd for a new life, I understood my upcoming paradox: wanting to be the best mother I could be, while recognizing that it may never feel good enough. My calling was to keep carrying on, moving forward despite the doubt and criticism I'd inevitably face. I needed to develop a bandwidth to tolerate the judgment so I would not be derailed by it. It reminded me of a classic Chris analogy: doubt (or any other troubling emotion) is like a fart in an elevator. Everyone knows it's there—it pervades the space—yet it doesn't prevent the elevator from working. Everyone still gets off at the right floor. This would be my work as a mother—notice that the elevator keeps working, and get off on the correct floor.

surrender

Toward the end of my pregnancy, inadvertently, Chris would jar me into yet another realization about motherhood. Chris needed a substitute for his class. In the past, he would have asked both Genevieve and me to take turns teaching for him, but this time he asked Genevieve. This news triggered me (hello, pregnancy hormones), and I called Chris in tears. "How could you do this?" I asked.

"It wasn't personal," he began. "I sensed into it and chose Genevieve. You are preparing to be a mother right now and that's more important."

I started to protest, insisting I was still willing and able to teach, but I sensed something else was going on. I was reaching an inevitable fork in the road. Until I had decided to have a child, teaching was my number one priority and pursuit. I aspired to one day call myself a Qigong master. This had become my identity, and now I was grasping onto it with all my might, despite—literally—growing evidence that my primary role was about to change. When I could be honest with myself, I knew Chris was right. I could viscerally feel the change presenting itself. I needed to step away from teaching for the time being. It did not necessarily need to be a permanent change, but for the moment I was being asked to let go, to surrender to a whole new me, though I can't say I fully did until my son was actually born. Birth has a way of making even the most stubborn people surrender on some level.

This identity shift—it's one of the most jarring parts of becoming a mom. Some aspects of your identity let go easily, but others hold on dearly, ready for a fight. In the end, I got hit over the head with a call for surrender that left no room for hanging on.

During my last month of pregnancy, I started to visit my midwife weekly. Everything had been going fine from a medical standpoint. The baby was growing, and so was I. I passed my gestational diabetes test, my blood pressure had remained low, and no protein showed up in my urine. Physically, I was slowing down significantly by the thirty-seventh week. I was out of breath, my ankles and legs were unrecognizably swollen, and my fingers were completely numb. Still, I knew I was fundamentally okay.

In preparation, with the meticulous futility of a mad scientist trying to control the weather, I created a birth plan, detailing every aspect of my son's arrival. The plan outlined that I would stay at home with Annette and Genevieve, doing Qigong exercises to control pain and coaxing full-blown labor to begin. I was hoping my experience would provide enough insight for me to develop a Qigong labor and birthing class in the future. When I got to the hospital, the instructions clearly explained, I wanted to avoid medical interventions as much as possible. I had spent my pregnancy researching medical intervention, a topic that had captivated me as an undergraduate earning a degree in medical anthropology. I was completely opposed to a cesarean birth unless my life or my son's life was at risk. I knew that even the simplest interventions often led to more and more invasive interventions, which inevitably resulted in an exceptionally high rate of C-sections. My birth plan also prescribed the ambiance and mood in the room: music, dimmed lights, and electric candles. I intended to squat throughout labor and give birth in this position rather than reclined in a bed. I wanted gravity's help, and I'd been squatting every day throughout my pregnancy to ward off back pain and to prepare me for what I saw as the most natural way to give birth. Either Vanya or Annette would catch the baby, who would be immediately placed on my chest for skin-to-skin contact, and the doctors would allow the umbilical cord to bleed out before clamping or cutting it.

Looking back now, many of these details seem absurd. But I had a vision, and I wanted to communicate it to my whole team. Despite the fact that a huge part of the birth class I'd attended had focused on letting go of expectations, I boldly (or maybe blindly) assumed I would get the birth I wanted. Hadn't I paid my dues getting pregnant? I was owed this wish.

But when I arrived at my midwife's office for my thirty-seven-week appointment, my plans came crashing to a halt. I tested my urine, weighed in, and took a seat in the waiting room, per usual. My urine tested normal, and my weight was on track. But when my midwife took my blood pressure, it was elevated for the first time. I'd run about 110 over 70 for most of my pregnancy, but now it was up around 135 over 85.

"Let's see whether your blood pressure resolves if you lay down on your left side," Claire, my midwife, suggested. It did, but she cautioned, "We need to keep an eye on this, but I think it's still okay. Just take it very easy this weekend. Lay down if you need to and just rest. Let's check on you on Monday."

I went home, vowing to take it much easier. I still had a huge list of things to do, but my body was telling me that I needed either to let go of the to-do list or enlist help. Friday afternoon, however, Claire called and reviewed my symptoms with me. She wasn't her usual calm self. "I'm worried about your blood pressure," she said. "I need you to call immediately if you feel faint or experience any nausea, headache, or swelling in your face, because it could mean you are developing preeclampsia." Her anxiety was contagious.

The next morning I awoke feeling nauseous and rushed into the bathroom, lightheaded, to puke. This freaked me out completely. I texted my midwife, not feeling bold enough to call her at 5:00 A.M. I crawled back in bed and tried to sleep. Within a few minutes, she called back, "You threw up?" she asked with an obvious note of concern. "How are you feeling otherwise?

"I feel fine," I responded.

"I think we should be cautious and go to the hospital," she decided. "I'll meet you in triage."

I hung up the phone, shaking. I rummaged around my room, packing an overnight bag. I couldn't remember the list of items suggested at our birth class, and I was kicking myself for not having packed a bag already. My roommates were still asleep, so I quietly waddled downstairs to the kitchen and scribbled a note. *I had to go to the hospital. Can you let the dogs out?*

In the darkness of pre-dawn, I drove myself to the hospital. It still felt too early to call anyone on my support team, and I assumed I'd be sent home again anyway, so I didn't want to bother anyone. But again my aloneness hit me as I drove the nearly empty streets.

When Claire arrived to meet me in triage, I was trembling with fear. My blood pressure was sky high. Remembering that stress was a huge factor in elevated blood pressure, before the next BP check I took a moment to calm my breathing and unclench my jaw. But for now, my midwife had reason to be concerned. She then did a pelvic exam to see if I had dilated at all. As she inserted her gloved hand into my body, I winced. I had heard about these exams, but no one warned me that I'd feel like I was being ripped sideways. I felt myself clamp down internally.

"You're not dilated at all," Claire reported. "Maybe at a 1.5 cm." With that she excused herself to consult the doctors in the practice.

Claire was a new midwife and only one of three midwives licensed to deliver babies at this hospital, under the supervision of an OB/GYN practice that specialized in high-risk pregnancies. She had explained many times that in the event of any complications, she would need to involve the doctors in the practice. She assured me that she would continue my care, with their supervision, for as long as she could before transferring me to their care entirely. I had never met any of these doctors.

I waited nervously in the cold, clinical triage area. Around me, monitors and alarms beeped constantly, reporting the stats of the other women in triage. We each had a few feet between our beds, with a curtain providing some modicum of privacy. Nurses came and went, attending to at least four women. I had no idea what to expect. My blood pressure still returned to normal range when I laid down or even just tilted the hospital bed. I had no protein in my urine, so I wasn't considered preeclampsic. Claire had explained that my puking was probably no big deal. "Usually when throwing up is associated with preeclampsia, you continue to throw up. An isolated incident was probably just indigestion," she had explained. Given these circumstances, plus the fact that I wasn't dilated at all, I assumed Claire would tell me to return home and rest.

But she returned with unexpected news, "I'm going to have you admitted, and I am transferring your care to the doctors." I gulped, not understanding why she was transferring my care straight out of the gates. "I will be there with you and can help advise you as a doula would do, but I will not be able to make any medical decisions anymore."

Claire explained that I could start with drugs or a foley bulb, which is an inflatable bulb inserted into the cervix to physically force it open, to induce labor. I initially agreed to a foley bulb at Claire's recommendation, but in the hour or two it took for me to be transferred to a room my gut had given me a loud and clear "No" about it. I told Claire I wanted to use the drugs instead, and she promised to inform the doctor of my decision.

But the doctor entered the room in a blaze of action, rolling a cart with medical instruments on it over to the bed. He gave me a perfunctory nod, before he sat down at the foot of the bed and asked me to spread my legs.

"Wait, I don't want to use the foley bulb," I said trying to hoist myself up on my arms so I could peer up over my enormous belly.

The doctor let out an exasperated sigh, "What? The order said you want a foley," he practically yelled at me.

I expected Claire to speak up for me, but she wasn't in the room. Suddenly I felt silly. Maybe the original plan had been best. "I had changed my mind and decided to start with the drugs instead. But okay, if you think the foley is best, I guess I'll do it." I couldn't point to any tangible reasons not to start with the foley, other than my amorphous gut instinct, which was still loudly protesting, but I wasn't about to explain that to this bristly doctor.

The procedure was a disaster. He could not get the bulb inserted, and I yelped in pain, my pelvis jumping a few feet off the bed. "You have a terrible yeast infection. Did you even know that?" he asked incredulously. "That's why I can't get the bulb in."

Claire, who had finally arrived back in the room, bristled at his comments, knowing this was an unlikely reason to have trouble inserting the bulb.

After his failed attempts, I began drugs to ripen my cervix and induce labor. Yet everything that could go wrong did, and labor never started. For one, I was in so much pain from the foley experience my insides were shaking. Each time I tried to pee, my body would shake and I'd start crying, unable to release the muscles necessary to pee. Almost twenty-four hours later, Chris, who had been traveling, arrived at the hospital and treated me for two hours, trying to calm my system down and induce labor. When he was done, I finally managed to pee, only to learn that the doctors were coming to check the progress of my cervix. Again, the exam sent me straight back into spasm.

Roughly forty-eight hours after I'd been admitted, I was showing no signs of dilation. A new nurse on shift came into my room to run my vitals. "Why are you here?" she asked innocently. "Your blood pressure isn't that high. I can ask the doctors if you can go home, since the induction isn't working." She returned to tell me the doctors had rejected the idea, but it was too late. The suggestion had taken hold. I was going home to relax and coax my baby to arrive, outside of the stress of the hospital. This caused a huge kerfuffle. The nurses suggested that if I left against medical advice my medical insurance would terminate—something I later learned was both untrue and illegal to suggest. The doctors threatened not to treat me when I returned to the hospital, and Claire was forced to recuse herself from my care completely, ending any contact with me whatsoever.

When I got home, I put myself on bed rest, spending hours in my zero gravity chair on my sunny porch, sipping juiced cucumber and eating other blood pressure reducing veggies. When I wasn't on my deck, I was floating in my bathtub filled with calming essential oils, or at the pool, since being immersed in water also lowers blood pressure. I borrowed a blood pressure cuff from a friend and monitored myself hourly. Chris treated me multiple times, trying to lower my blood pressure and induce labor. For the first week and a half of my home treatment, my blood pressure was lower than at the hospital, and it remained completely normal if I was laying down. Although my entire focus was on staying calm and relaxed, it was also a harrowing week of anticipating the unknown.

After ten days at home, my blood pressure started to climb. I called the hospital to talk to the midwife on duty, who assured me I could work with the midwife team as long as possible and start with drugs before attempting another foley bulb. With my primary concerns addressed, I hauled my carefully-packed hospital bag to the car and drove myself to the hospital once again. There I met Hannah, a wonderful and loving doula, who would assist me day and night, advocating for my preferences and keeping me company when my friends and birth team were unavailable.

Six days later, two doctors stood at the foot of my bed strongly encouraging me to agree to a cesarean section before they went off-shift. They had been trying to induce labor since I had admitted myself into the hospital, and I had barely even a single labor contraction. My blood pressure was still normal if I was lying down, and the baby had never been in distress, so up to this point I had refused a C-section. But I was bumping up against hospital policy that only allows women to be induced for four days. Period. As far as I could tell, it was as much a financial decision as it was related to medical necessity. These two doctors, with whom I had developed a good rapport over the past several days, warned that if I didn't let them operate, the next doctor on shift would be unkind. They even insinuated that the other doctor was so mad at me for not previously having agreed to a C-section that she would not do a good job on the surgery.

"Trust me. You do not want her operating on you," one of the doctors explained.

I relented to the surgery I'd been fighting for a week to avoid. My son was born healthy at 5:57 A.M. on April 3, his due date.

Although the doctors do not allow skin-to-skin contact in the operating room, they bundled my Aiden into a little burrito and held him up near my face. In what felt like a miracle, he kissed my cheek. I held back sobs of joy, worried that my shaking body would impede the doctors working diligently to sew me back up.

Then Aiden was whisked out of the freezing cold operating room into the loving arms of Annette, who was so dedicated to skin-to-skin contact that she ripped off her shirt, only to be reprimanded by the nurses.

Forty-five minutes later, Aiden and I were reunited. Through my drugged haze, I held him close, never wanting to let him go again. We spent those first few days in the hospital, with friends taking rotating shifts to help me lift Aiden, since I couldn't even get out of bed.

Jane and Leonardo, who had been traveling to New York, extended their trip and stopped through the Bay Area to visit. By coincidence they arrived on Aiden's birthday, and it was a joy to have them.

How do you describe what it's like finally to welcome the baby you worked so hard to bring into the world? Our first few weeks were blissful in so many ways. The support I had once worried I wouldn't have showed up in force. Friends and family brought food for several weeks, and for even longer my neighbor checked before she went to the grocery store to ask if I needed anything. Other friends stepped up to walk my dogs and help with household chores. Their assistance allowed me to nestle into a bubble with Aiden, marveling over the simple fact of his existence, this perfect being who had arrived in my life after so much struggle. I joked with friends that I feared I'd never get out of my chair again. I was a milk factory, first and foremost, and that seemed to occupy every waking (and sleeping) moment. But in truth, this was exactly what I had longed for, the role I had once feared I would never be able to fill.

For all the drama of his arrival, Aiden himself showed up comfortable and content. While other moms struggled with colicky babies or babies who just could not be soothed, rarely did I experience a moment when I could not provide what Aiden needed in order to be at peace. Perhaps I was granted a free pass for the difficulties I'd endured getting to this place?

Though Aiden appeared unfazed by his birth, I struggled to integrate the experience. As grateful as I was that my beautiful bundle arrived safe and sound, I was in a state of shock about my birth experience, heartbroken that I did not have the birth I had expected. The physical aftermath of the C-section complicated my early weeks as a mother. Every time I tried to sit up or roll over, it felt like someone was ripping my sutures apart stitch by stitch. Every time I nursed Aiden, I struggled to position him without feeling like someone was sawing my stomach open. As a single mom, trying to care for a newborn while recovering, physically and emotionally, from a C-section was like Motherhood Bootcamp.

I turned to Chris to help me put things in perspective.

"You don't want to bathe your newborn child in your anger about the birth," he cautioned, encouraging me to move forward as quickly as possible. "This is a special time that you don't want to miss because you are still upset about how he was born."

But I *was* upset. I felt robbed of the birth I had wanted.

"You did your best and tried everything in your power, which you needed to do," Chris continued. "From what I can tell, having a C-section was the safest possible thing for you and the baby."

I took this to heart, examining how I might be able to see the situation differently. First and foremost, I had a healthy baby—a big baby, weighing in at nine pounds twelve ounces, with a ninety-eighth percentile head. I understood how this might not have been kind to my small body. Maybe someone had been looking out for me? Keeping me safe? Once again, I could see how my expectations—particularly my idea that I could control my birth experience with a carefully detailed birth plan—had set me up for suffering.

To say my birth did not live up to my dreams would be an enormous understatement. In fact, I was so opposed to C-sections that if someone had told me before getting pregnant that I would need one, it's possible that I would not have had a baby. The surgery cuts through the dantien, the energetic center of the body, and I feared how this would affect both my Qigong practice and my health. For so many reasons, accepting this outcome would be a tall order. Then again, nothing about becoming a mother had gone according to plan. When first presented with the idea of having a baby alone I rejected it, and when told to use an egg donor, again I rejected it. Yet here I was nesting with my gorgeous, healthy, perfect son, with no regrets about those decisions, with a deep knowing that the whole fraught journey—even the C-section—had been worth it. In the end, more than any experience to date, giving birth ripped the idea of control out of my hands, requiring me to surrender. Being cut open then producing sustenance for my child from my wrecked body—it was like being told, "Welcome to motherhood. Your life, your body, your identity, and your notion of control are gone! Get used to it!" I did. I got used to it. Because that's what mothers do: we step up for our children, over and over again. I'd earned my Motherhood badge, and I was proud of it.

In addition to relinquishing control, I could feel parenthood calling me to surrender my current identity and transform into a different woman—a mother. I was well accustomed to shifting identities and the practice of reevaluating who I thought I was. A large part of Qigong practice centers around the ability to drop the body, to experience a sensation of disappearing into the energetic channels, shattering into hundreds of points of light, morphing into other shapes. The possibilities are endless, but the key is the ability to challenge one's perception, and one's firmly held beliefs about self. As Chris explains it, "It's easy to rigidify around a notion of yourself that has nothing to do with your essence. If you can drop your identity and put yourself down, over and over, you can begin to recognize your essence." Not only had I put my idea of myself down in Qigong class numerous times, but I'd been forced to put down my life as a lawyer, I'd shattered my expectations of how I was supposed become a mother, I'd put my identity as an aspiring Qigong master on the back burner, and I'd been blindsided by how my son was born. Could I do it again? Release the self I knew and welcome this transformation?

Back when I'd asked Chris if he thought I was pregnant, he'd told me I was completely different, that I'd dumped a whole pile of unhealthy behaviors in preparation for becoming a mother. At the time, I had no idea what he was talking about, but now, in every cell of my body I knew what he'd meant. I had gone through an impossibly powerful rite of passage, emerging into my nurturing, loving essence, the mother I had dreamed of being.

In fact, the transformation had already happened. I could fight it, or I could surrender into being the best mother I could to this beloved baby. I chose the latter. More than ever, I felt prepared to embrace the fluidity of life and my place within it.

epilogue

"Mama, there's a fire. I need to put it out. You stay here where it's safe," Aiden says, holding up his hand to tell me to stop moving as he runs off with a fake firehose in hand. Moments later he returns, peeling off his fire hat and fire suit. "The fire is out," he proclaims. "Now it is time for fire lunch. You sit here while I make us lunch."

My heart melts, and I sit down as instructed. I am at once bored to tears of this game and overcome with pride and joy. My son has been obsessed with firefighters for over a year now, and he stages rescues all day long, always protecting me, making sure I'm safe.

Admittedly, life is a little crazy. I am sleep deprived beyond measure. For a few hours a day, my son goes to daycare, and I frantically work, walk my dogs, prepare food for us, and run my business in that short time. If I'm lucky, he takes an afternoon nap. Afterwards, we head off to the park or the fire station, a visit we make at least once a week. Once I've put Aiden down for the night, I pull out my computer and work some more. Sometimes I wonder how I am surviving, yet I am the happiest I have ever been. My life feels full, complete, and whole. The struggles I went through have faded into the background, an insignificant price to pay for the unparalleled experience of motherhood. Ten years ago, I wouldn't have written the script of my life this way, but now that I am living it, it feels perfect. Given the chance, I wouldn't change a thing.

I never contemplate dating. I can't quite fathom how to get dressed up and out the door for something social, and the thought of wasting money on babysitting for what could be a bad date? It's nerve wracking. But more than that, I have no desire. My heart is cracked open by the love of my son every day. I relish in our closeness, and for now it feels natural to focus my time and energy there. I can't imagine it any other way.

It turned out my quest for pregnancy served as a training ground for motherhood. Throughout the hopes and disappointments, the freak outs and returns to clarity, I learned the fundamentals of motherhood. I dissolved self-doubt and hatred, learned how to be satisfied with doing my best, recognized that nothing except love makes sense, realized that self-doubt and criticism are a choice and a call to return home to my essence, and most importantly I learned to let go of the need to control the outcome, instead finding the gifts in any outcome.

Frankly, I don't have time to indulge in the neuroses that used to spin me for days. If insecurity or anxiety arises, I drop it and keep moving forward in service of my son. In this way, motherhood—my dedication to showing up for my son and, let's be honest, the utter lack of free time—has given me a rudder. I rarely lose my bearings, in large part because of the healing work I have done, but also because I simply can't. I have a clear vision of what's right for me and my son, and I don't get pushed off course.

In fact, sometimes I'm so focused on moving us through our days that I don't notice all I'm doing until someone holds up a mirror for me. Like one morning, when my son was about two years old, I was at a café, struggling to put a lid on my coffee and carry my food order, wallet, car keys, *and* my son all out the door at the same time. A woman in the coffee shop overheard me muttering to my son, "Let's see if we can do this."

She said, "Girlfriend, of course you can do it — you're a mom, right? That's what we do, Mama. We get it done!"

"Damn straight," I replied, maybe a little too enthusiastically, as I fumbled to set down my coffee and pastry so I could give her a high-five, with my son balanced on my hip. Tears welled as I recognized all that I do on my own: running a business, writing a book, maintaining my home, caring for two dogs, raising my son, managing my tenants — the list goes on. Yes, I'm doing it all alone. But the silver lining? This feeling that I can handle *anything*. That's right, Mama, I get it done.

Though the prospect of forgoing a genetic connection to my future child had concerned me, and at times I feared that it might impact our bond, it hasn't. The other day, as I was serving him dinner, Aiden asked, "Mama, will you bring your chair and talk to me while I eat?" After I pulled up my itty bitty toddler chair to join him, he announced, "I'll go first. Um . . . today I played with my friends and made lunch for everyone in the kitchen after I rescued a kitten from a tree. Okay, now your turn. You talk to me now." Of course, my heart broke open for the hundredth time that day as I imagined our years to come, sitting down at dinner to tell each other about our days.

The love I feel for Aiden is exactly what mothers describe: immense, bigger than I could have fathomed. Further, whether Aiden carries my genes or not has become completely irrelevant to me. I love this child with all my heart, body, and soul. With that love comes a certainty that he is exactly the child I was meant to have. We feel completely, exquisitely, perfectly in sync. There is no doubt that he is 100 percent mine. Now that Aiden is here, I can't believe I ever agonized over the decision to use an egg donor. When I look back on my path, my only regret is that I didn't take the leap sooner. I wish I could grab every woman contemplating single motherhood or the use of an egg donor and tell her, "You won't regret it. In fact, when your child arrives, you won't believe how irrelevant it seems."

My experience getting pregnant has completely reshaped my life, reconnecting me to my passion for women's reproductive rights and all things maternal. It's strange, maybe even ironic, that my life has come completely full circle, making me into a walking, breathing example of women's reproductive rights and bioethics. I've even considered dusting off my law degree to help perspective parents with donor agreements and policies surrounding advanced reproductive technologies and alternative family structures.

I've also shifted my coaching and Embodied Clarity Approach to focus on women who want to become mothers, no matter what it takes. After trudging through the trenches, figuring it all out on my own; after debating whether I'd be able to make it work as a single mother; after doing extensive research on alternative therapies for fertility enhancement, cycle tracking, and options for insemination both at home and at the fertility clinic; after navigating sperm banks; after weighing the options available, including fresh versus frozen eggs, embryo adoption, adoption, egg donation, and fertility services abroad; after learning so many lessons the hard way, I am sharing my information and wisdom. I guide and mentor women who are contemplating single motherhood, seeking help with fertility and egg donation, or raising donor-conceived children. In addition to supporting my clients through the emotional ups and downs, and the dizzying information and logistics, I help my clients cultivate the love, courage, and tenacity it takes to conceive and raise a child through unconventional means. I help them find their unique, no-regrets paths to motherhood, so they can get down to being their own badass mama selves.

You can find more information about my coaching services, courses, and support communities at:
www.motherhoodreimagined.com

acknowledgements

This book would not have been possible without the tireless help of Brooke Warner an incredible editor and master at helping tease out the meaning and intention of my words. Thank you to Roy Carlisle for planting the seed that my story was worthy of being a book and encouraging me to write in the first place. And to my friends and incredible support network for listening to me talk about working on my book for the last several years, and supporting and encouraging me to continue.

Many, but not all, of the names have been changed in this book to protect the privacy of the individuals mentioned.

about the author

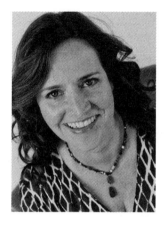

Sarah Kowalski, Esq., is a fertility doula, family building coach, postpartum doula, and author, as well as the founder of Motherhood Reimagined. She is a regular contributor to YourTango.com, and ChoiceMoms.org as well as a Resource Guide and Contributing Author at ESME.com. As a single mother by choice who conceived her son via sperm and egg donors, she provides coaching, e-courses and support groups for women who are contemplating single motherhood, having fertility issues, raising donor-conceived children, or navigating life as single mothers. Kowalski has a BA from UC Berkeley, and she graduated magna cum laude from Santa Clara University Law School in 1998. She left the practice of law to pursue her interests in alternative healing and the mind/body connection by becoming a Guild-Certified Feldenkrais Practitioner, Qigong instructor, and Certified Integral Coach.

Author photo © Reenie Raschke

selected titles from she writes press

She Writes Press is an independent publishing
company founded to serve women writers everywhere.
Visit us at www.shewritespress.com.

The Doctor and The Stork: A Memoir of Modern Medical Baby-making by K.K. Goldberg. $16.95, 978-1-63152-830-9. A mother's compelling story of her post-IVF, high-risk pregnancy with twins—the very definition of a modern medical babymaking experience.

Expecting Sunshine: A Journey of Grief, Healing, and Pregnancy after Loss by Alexis Marie Chute. $16.95, 978-1-63152-174-4. A mother's inspiring story of surviving pregnancy following the death of one of her children at birth.

A Leg to Stand On: An Amputee's Walk into Motherhood by Colleen Haggerty. $16.95, 978-1-63152-923-8. Haggerty's candid story of how she overcame the pain of losing a leg at seventeen—and of terminating two pregnancies as a young woman—and went on to become a mother, despite her fears.

Breathe: A Memoir of Motherhood, Grief, and Family Conflict by Kelly Kittel. $16.95, 978-1-938314-78-0. A mother's heartbreaking account of losing two sons in the span of nine months—and learning, despite all the obstacles in her way, to find joy in life again.

Make a Wish for Me: A Mother's Memoir by LeeAndra Chergey. $16.95, 978-1-63152-828-6. A life-changing diagnosis teaches a family that where's there is love there is hope—and that being "normal" is not nearly as important as providing your child with a life full of joy, love, and acceptance.

Three Minus One: Parents' Stories of Love & Loss edited by Sean Hanish and Brooke Warner. $17.95, 978-1-938314-80-3. A collection of stories and artwork by parents who have suffered child loss that offers insight into this unique and devastating experience.

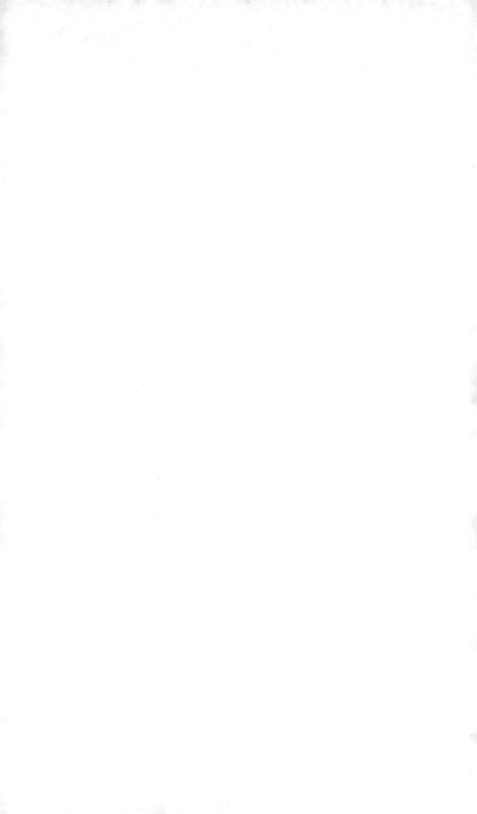